Ethnicity
in Social
Group Work
Practice

The *Social Work with Groups* series

Series Editors: Catherine P. Papell and Beulah Rothman

Ethnicity in Social Group Work Practice

Larry E. Davis
Guest Editor

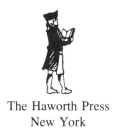

The Haworth Press
New York

Ethnicity in Social Group Work Practice has also been published as *Social Work with Groups*, Volume 7, Number 3, Fall 1984.

The Haworth Press, Inc., 28 East 22 Street, New York, NY 10010

Library of Congress Cataloging in Publication Data
Main entry under title:

Ethnicity in social group work practice.

   Also published as v. 7, no. 3 of: Social work with groups.
   Includes bibliographical references.
   1. Social work with minorities—United States—Addresses, essays, lectures.   2. Social group work—Addresses, essays, lectures.   I. Davis, Larry E.
HV3176.E84   1984   362.8'4   84-6628
ISBN 0-86656-323-7

Ethnicity in Social Group
Work Practice

Social Work with Groups
Volume 7, Number 3

CONTENTS

JUDITH B. LEE, DSW, *School of Social Work, New York University, New York, New York*

BARUCH LEVINE, PhD, *Jane Addams College of Social Work, University of Illinois, and private practice, Chicago*

HENRY W. MAIER, PhD, *School of Social Work, University of Washington, Seattle*

RUTH R. MIDDLEMAN, EdD, *Raymond A. Kent School of Social Work, University of Louisville, Kentucky*

HELEN NORTHEN, PhD, *School of Social Work, University of Southern California, Los Angeles*

RUBY B. PERNELL, DSW, *School of Applied Social Sciences, Case Western Reserve University, Cleveland*

HELEN PHILLIPS, DSW, *School of Social Work, University of Pennsylvania, Philadelphia*

HERMAN RESNICK, PhD, *School of Social Work, University of Washington, Seattle*

SHELDON ROSE, PhD, *School of Social Work, University of Wisconsin, Madison*

JANICE H. SCHOPLER, MSW, *School of Social Work, University of North Carolina, Chapel Hill*

LAWRENCE SHULMAN, EdD, *School of Social Work, University of British Columbia, Vancouver, Canada*

MARY LOUISE SOMERS, DSW, *School of Social Service Administration, University of Chicago*

EMANUEL TROPP, MSSW, *School of Social Work, Virginia Commonwealth University, Richmond*

ROBERT VINTER, PhD, *School of Social Work, University of Michigan, Ann Arbor*

CELIA B. WEISMAN, DSW, *Wurzweiler School of Social Work, Yeshiva University, New York*

GERTRUDE WILSON, MA, *University of California, Berkeley*

EDITORIAL

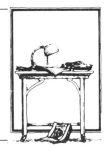

This issue of *Social Work with Groups* is a testimonial to professional commitment to a pluralistic, multi-ethnic society. In direct opposition to the "melting pot," it heightens awareness and understanding of the needs and resources of minority ethnic groups of color and presents the contribution that social work with groups can make to the strengthening of both ethnic and universal identity so necessary in our contemporary society. Formulations of pluralism, ethnic identity and differentiation rather than assimilation, are addressed in the context of professional practice and concerns. The contributors who have authored these papers take us inside the worlds of differing ethnic groups, providing insights that can affect our purposes and actions as practitioners.

From our reading of the papers we believe that group workers will find it possible to meet the challenge. They will be able to translate traditional values and skills in working with people with special needs shaped by their cultural experiences. From our readings we also know that one is confronted with a profound experience in self-awareness as one sees one's own cultural world in juxtaposition to the several different minority groups. The varied ways that culture prescribes and patterns how one goes about the business of living is vividly presented in this collection of papers. The guidelines for practice with ethnic groups will be useful to all social workers but will require examination anew of one's own identity in relation to clients' strivings to fulfull theirs.

These articles once again demonstrate the value of social group

1

work in its service to people in coping with alienation and loneliness in an unfamiliar overwhelming, contradictory and often unhospitable world. It becomes clear in the content of these articles how the small group can become the primary means by which the individual and the larger ethnic community are reconciled. The abstraction of our late colleague, William Schwartz, regarding the small group's mediating function between individual and societal need is brought to life. For the individual of color two worlds exists, the normal culture for instrumental security and survival, and the ethnic culture for affective and nurturing supports. How the small group, in a unique and complex way, links the person with both the ethnic community and the larger culture is represented here. In these papers the ideology and methodology of social group work meets the new demand, placing the process in a transcultural perspective. Group work serves a two-fold function, strengthening identity with one's heritage, and enabling emergence into the dominant world.

From a mental health perspective the small group, in acting as a conduit between the ethnic and the dominant communities offers belonging and counters alienation. Identification with the ethnic community, can be a force in sustaining and rebuilding interpersonal security and self-realization. These papers also illuminate how it is possible to facilitate coping with the stress of belonging to two worlds. Perhaps ethnic identity or its counterpart is necessary in a mass society which fails to adequately provide for interpersonal development needs and satisfactions.

The presentation of the ethnic community in these papers transcends physical boundaries and sets forth the psychological entity of community as a reality in determining behavior and development. Through group work not only can the individual be enriched, but the ethnic community is restored legitimately as a part of the pluralistic whole. Thus group work can continue to participate in the development of a more just society.

The editors of this journal acknowledge the debt owed to our guest editor, Dr. Larry Davis, for bringing together this outstanding collection of papers. The continuing consideration of ethnicity as an issue in social work practice with groups and as a vital aspect of the social work profession's societal mission can be pursued with new direction and energy because of the standard of theoretical discussion and practice achieved in these papers.

CP
BR

GUEST EDITORIAL

THE SIGNIFICANCE OF COLOR

Eighty years ago, W.E.B. Dubois predicted that the problem of the twentieth century would be the problem of color. Since that time, numerous theories have been put forth in an attempt to explain the causes of America's social ills. However, despite the many factors which affect individual Americans—such as income, education, gender and age, etc.—none has as clearly nor as consistently demonstrated its potency as has skin color. Color remains one of the best predictors of a population being "at risk." Indeed, an individual's skin is our best predictor of the quality of life experiences which he or she, despite other mediating factors, is likely to encounter. It is for this reason that we have elected to focus the attention of this special issue exclusively upon group work with ethnic groups of color. Such a focus is not to suggest that ethnicity as circumscribed by culture and/or language, is not also a salient factor and hence, a strong predictor of life events—we believe that it is. However, we do wish to emphasize the preeminence of skin color, as it so often serves to demarcate those who are in the greatest need of services frequently provided by group workers.

THE CHALLENGE TO GROUP WORK

Demographers predict that the number of non-white minorities will increase from their 1980 proportion of approximately 17 percent to approximately 30 percent of the American populace by the year 2000. There are also indications, such as high birth rates and low levels of employable skills, that a disproportionate number of persons of color will be "at risk" and, hence, in need of some sort of social service. Moreover, there are strong indications that monies available to hire additional social service personnel will—if the present economic and political atmosphere prevails—fall far behind the need for service delivery.

In anticipation of these three occurrences—(1) disproportionate growth in non-white minority groups, (2) corresponding dispro-portionate growth in their need for social services, and (3) relative decline in resources to hire persons to deliver services to those in need it would seem reasonable to expect that greater reliance will have to be made on group work as a means of service delivery. If so, all types of treatment groups composed entirely or in part of non-white minorities will become the rule more frequently than the exception.

The above scenario presents a prodigious challenge to those who teach and practice group work. Basically, the challenge has two foci. First, due to the strong possibility of an increased need for social services and relatively fewer personnel to provide it, social work must produce greater numbers of practitioners who are trained to deliver social services via the small group. That is, because the helping professions will be called upon to do more for greater numbers of individuals with relatively fewer numbers with which to do it, they must rely on greater numbers of those who practice, to do so with groups. Therefore, we encourage those who are at the helms of direct service curricula to advocate greater resource allocation to the training of group workers.

Second, because we anticipate that the largest growth in the need for services will be among members of non-white minority groups, those teaching and practicing group work must be better informed regarding group work with non-white populations. This special issue on ethnicity is principally an attempt to address this concern. Therefore, America's four largest non-white populations have been selected for consideration here: American Indians, Asians, Hispan-ics, and Blacks. Each of the articles included in this issue attempts to increase the reader's understanding of group work practice with one of these minority groups of color. Each article has attempted to ac-complish at least two goals: (1) to enlighten practitioners who have little familiarity with the specific racial groups under discussion about some of the basic ingredients of group work with these minor-ity groups, and (2) to enlighten further those who already have exist-ing knowledge of group work with particular minority groups. Moreover, it is our hope that issues addressed in these articles will serve to assist all practitioners who lead groups which contain mem-bers whose color and/or ethnicity differs from that of their own.

There are already indications, based on the number of articles being published, that the use of group work with minorities of color is in a period of growth. And, in view of the projected racial demographics, there is little reason to expect that this rate of group work practice with persons of color will decline. Therefore, the question before us is not will persons of color be seen in groups, but rather will the practitioners leading those groups be sufficiently skilled and knowledgeable about group work with ethnic minorities of color to lead them effectively. It is hoped that the wide assortment of practice issues and clinical perspectives presented in this issue will serve to better prepare those group practitioners who work with non-whites to do so with greater sensitivity and skill.

* * *

I want to thank the following individuals who served as members of the review committee for this special issue on ethnicity and group work. Their critical evaluations and comments on the great many papers, which were submitted for review, enhanced appreciably the overall quality of this issue.

Pallassana Balgopal
School of Social Work
University of Illinois
   at Urbana Champaign
Urbana, Illinois

Leon Chestang
School of Social Work
Wayne State University
Detroit, Michigan

Melvin Delgado
School of Social Work
Boston University
Boston, Massachusetts

Ronald Feldman
George Warren Brown
   School of Social Work
Washington University
St. Louis, Missouri

John Gallegos
School of Social Work
   College of Human Services
San Diego State University
San Diego, California

Harriet McAdoo
School of Social Work
Howard University
Washington, D.C.

Larry E. Davis
George Warren Brown
School of Social Work
Washington University

Group Work Practice with American Indians

E. Daniel Edwards
Margie E. Edwards

ABSTRACT. This paper discusses ways in which social group work can be implemented in behalf of American Indian clientele. Social workers should be aware of the value that American Indians have placed on the use of groups within their own culture, and the importance of understanding the impact of American Indian culture on each individual American Indian client and tribal group. A number of current issues facing American Indian people are identified. Suggestions are offered for consideration in planning specific group experiences.

Group work is becoming the treatment of choice for a number of agencies with programs serving American Indians. The variety and extent of group intervention is growing as American Indian people are finding satisfaction in sharing concerns, and addressing problems in group efforts. Many American Indians have enjoyed participation in cultural group activities and are able to transfer some of these positive feelings to the group experiences offered by social group workers.

THE PLACE OF GROUPS IN AMERICAN INDIAN CULTURE

American Indian culture traditionally has focused on a variety of group activities which have brought families, clans, and tribal groups together for social, cultural, and religious activities. Human

E. Daniel Edwards, DSW is an Associate Professor with the Graduate School of Social Work, University of Utah. He is a Yurok Indian from northern California, and is Director of the University of Utah's American Indian Social Work Career Training Program. Margie E. Edwards, PhD is a Professor with the Graduate School of Social Work, University of Utah. She is a former coordinator of the American Indian Social Work Career Training Program.
Requests for reprints may be addressed to the authors at the Graduate School of Social Work, University of Utah, Salt Lake City, UH 84112.

7

growth and development experiences are often celebrated with group activities which involve family and clan members. In some tribal groups, the occasion of a baby's first smile or laughter is cause for group celebration, and family and clan members gather to wish a happy and joyful existence for the infant. ''Rites of passage'' are celebrated in some tribal groups with extended family and clan participation. Marriage ceremonies bring friends and family together to honor the new bride and groom and to offer advice and counsel to promote a successful and happy marital union. Special seasons of the year or events related to planting and harvesting are celebrated with group activity in the form of games, dances, music, contests, and group interaction. Many of these activities are similar, but there is considerable uniqueness with each individual tribal group.

THE IMPORTANCE OF UNDERSTANDING "CULTURE" IN WORKING WITH AMERICAN INDIANS

Each of the many individual tribal groups is unique in many respects. It is also important to understand the uniqueness of each American Indian person. Although many stereotypes persist regarding American Indian children, adults, and older people, the individuality of each American Indian person is widely respected among most American Indian tribal groups. This uniqueness must also be respected by social workers.

Family ties, bonds, and expectations also vary considerably among each of the more than 480 tribal groups in the United States today. Some tribal groups emphasize strong extended family ties. Many tribes promote a matriarchal or patriarchal family structure. Some families maintain strong traditional ties to their culture and reservation or Indian lands. Many American Indians have spent considerable time in off-reservation locales—urban areas, in the armed service, in employment settings, and in educational settings. All of these experiences have influenced the lives of American Indian people and the extent of their cultural ties.

A large number of American Indian tribal groups emphasize the importance of maintaining their tribal languages. Tribal customs among these groups are equally emphasized. Other tribal groups encourage fluency in Indian languages and in the English language. Some tribal groups are relatively small and have lost much of their tribal language and cultural ties. Among those American Indian people where culture and tradition have been stressed, there is extensive identification and respect for Indian values and customs. The extent of such identification should be evaluated carefully in working with American Indian people.

Studying and learning about American Indian culture can be a fascinating and rewarding experience for Indian and non-Indian social workers. Such a study often leads to an appreciation of the cultural heritage of American Indian people and an enhanced awareness of the many issues facing American Indian people today. This understanding can promote identification of issues toward which social workers could be giving attention in their work with American Indian people.

CURRENT ISSUES FACING AMERICAN INDIAN PEOPLE

There are a number of important issues facing American Indian people today. Social workers should be aware of these concerns as they often provide tangible evidence of social and cultural needs, as well as opportunities for social work intervention to address these issues. Cultural identification is an example of such a concern. Many American Indian people are expressing an interest in becoming more involved with American Indian programs, politics, and cultural activities. Recreational and cultural activities are being promoted in both reservation and urban settings. Indian people are openly participating in American Indian games and contests, pow-wows and dances, recreational tournaments, and cultural competition. Young people are being encouraged to develop their cultural skills. Older people are enjoying participation in games and contest events which have been important to them since their youth. As social workers become aware of such programs, appropriate referrals can be made to available resources. Where there are fewer opportunities for cultural involvement, social workers may provide leadership in initiating and supporting program development.

The urbanization of American Indians is being recognized as an issue to which attention should be given by American Indian people. Thornton, Sandefur, and Grasmich (1982) have identified some of the social changes which have resulted from the movement of American Indian people to urban areas. This movement began in the late 1940s, after World War II, and has continued to develop. Many

American Indian people move to urban areas because of experiences they have had in the military. They are often seeking employment opportunities. Government "relocation and training programs" encouraged American Indian people to receive training and accept employment in urban areas. This movement has, however, not been without its impact. Distance has affected the extent of opportunities for extended family involvement and participation in tribal activities. Many American Indian people have found it necessary to maintain continued close contact with family on reservations in order to promote their children's identification with American Indian culture. There are often considerable "pulls" to reservations from older American Indian people and particularly parents, uncles and aunts, and grandparents. Some American Indian people have not adjusted well to urbanization and have experienced problems with alcoholism, loneliness, and alienation in an urban setting. The influx of American Indian people to urban settings has also fostered development of American Indian centers, health programs, and multitribal activities as American Indian people have banded together to promote continued participation in cultural and social activities. Many of the needs of urban American Indian people could be addressed through provision of social work services, and particularly group services. The initiation of such programs would facilitate adjustment to urban settings while capitalizing on cultural strengths and activities.

The development of American Indian leadership is also an important issue. Many American Indian tribal groups have promoted the need for "self-determination" among their Indian people. This recognized need has led to the involvement of American Indian men and women in leadership positions. Leadership development has been fostered through training programs, involvement of American Indians in higher education programs, and "on-the-job training." Continued leadership development is recommended for Indian youth and adults and could be fostered through appropriate social work planning and intervention.

Unemployment continues to impact upon American Indian people today. Other economic development issues are also topics of concern among American Indians. Attention to these issues may be facilitated through the efforts of a social group worker through a task group or community organization approach.

Stereotyping of American Indian people persists in our society. Arlene B. Hirschfelder (1982) has been successful in identifying a variety of materials that promote the correction of offending images of American Indians (pp. 269-296). These materials could be valuable to American Indian youth and older people, as well as to non-Indians in heightening awareness of stereotypes which persist today—another area in which social work could be involved. Educational issues continue to confront American Indian people in public schools, boarding schools, higher education programs, and adult education programs. Adult education programs may be helpful in addressing some additional issues which impact upon older American Indian people today. Many educational settings are utilizing social workers in providing direct services to clientele as well as in program development and planning capacities.

Much has been written about the problems of American Indian people. However, there are movements afoot to address the strengths as well as the stresses of American Indian individuals and families. A recent American Indian conference (1980) addressed the importance of supporting and strengthening Indian families (p. iii). Other efforts are being encouraged to address similar topics. Social work intervention in this area could capitalize on identification and mobilization of resources of American Indian people as well as prevention of problematic behaviors through enhancement of individual and tribal strengths.

Social workers have been helpful in identifying a variety of issues facing the American Indian people with whom they work. Creative employment of group approaches has been successful in addressing many of these problems. Several structural issues should be considered in planning appropriate group experiences for American Indian people. A discussion of this topic follows.

GROUP FORMATION AND PLANNING ISSUES

Many American Indian social workers are currently employed in agencies serving Native American people. These social workers provide American Indian clientele with models of those who have successfully encountered and achieved in higher educational systems today. However, a number of non-Indian social workers are also effective in their work with American Indian clientele. Geraldine Youngman and Margaret Sandonegei (1979) have identified some leader behaviors which will facilitate developing relationships with American Indian children. These behaviors are equally important for American Indian and non-Indian social workers and include the necessity of patience in establishing client/worker relationships. The importance of assessing and understanding the verbal skills of the American Indian client is also stressed by these authors as is the ability to communicate the sincerity of the helping person. Social workers should avoid asking too many personal questions too early in the professional relationship. In addition to these considerations, it is important for social workers to understand the individual client's perception of the importance of his/her independence. Many American Indian tribal groups reinforce the value of each individual American Indian person. Each person is allowed the freedom to make personal decisions. Others respect individual decisions even though they may, at times, not agree with the choices the person has made. A strong sense of responsibility also accompanies this independence value. Many American Indian people see themselves as responsible for making their own decisions, and they may, therefore, resist the helping relationship offered by the social worker.

Another value of many American Indians is their respect for the privacy of others. It is important that American Indians not speak for other American Indian people, including mates, children, extended family members, and certainly not other tribal members. It may, therefore, be inappropriate for Indian people to assess the feelings of their significant others.

Another important value of American Indian people is that of bringing honor and respect to themselves, their tribal group and their family. This expectation should be addressed realistically (bragging and exaggerations are equally frowned upon). It is also equally crucial that American Indians not embarrass themselves or others. Seeking professional help may imply an inability to handle one's own problems, and, therefore, bring some embarrassment upon themselves or other family members. Some of these values will often be in conflict with the reaching out efforts of social workers, and may be better understood within the cultural context of an American Indian person's identification.

Co-leading of American Indian groups is often a rewarding and satisfying worker relationship, not only for the social workers, but for many American Indian clientele. With a male and female co-worker structure, it may be easier for some clients to identify with males, and some to identify with females, as often is the case in non-Indian social work intervention. Also, an Indian social worker and a non-Indian social worker may present opportunities to address Indian and non-Indian issues which impact upon the American Indian client. Co-leaders may also bring divergent strengths, background experiences, values, ideas, and feelings to the group experience. One American Indian alcoholism group is being led by an recovering Indian alcoholic and a non-Indian social drinker. The leaders model the respect they hold for each other, and they also express different experiences and viewpoints about experiences with alcohol.

STRUCTURING THE GROUP FOR GOAL ATTAINMENT

Structuring the group for goal attainment is an important consideration. Some groups may meet for short-term experiences while others require long-term intervention. Issues related to appropriate settings and group meeting days and times are important issues which should be addressed to facilitate the attainment of the group's purposes and goals. The more American Indian clientele can be involved in such decision making, the greater the likelihood of success for the group experience.

A group's potential success will be enhanced when goals and purposes are clearly defined for both the group and individual members. When purposes are well defined, group members will be more aware of the objectives to which they are committing themselves. They will also have a framework from which to establish their own individual goals. A young adult alcoholism group may have the following purpose: to help members with drinking problems change their attitudes and behaviors. Objectives could relate to discussion of (1) healthy and unhealthy drinking attitudes, (2) facts and myths about alcohol, (3) early warning signs of alcohol addiction, (4) phases of alcoholism, (5) individual responsibility and problem solving and decision-making skills, (6) alternatives to alcohol use in solving problems and handling feelings, and (7) awareness of resources to assist members.

Individual goals for members of a young adult alcoholism group may include the following: (1) admitting the extent of an individual's drinking problem; (2) identifying antecedents to drinking behaviors; (3) identifying sources of support which could be helpful in overcoming drinking problems such as non-drinking friends and family members, Alcoholics Anonymous, alcoholism treatment and recovery facilities; (4) identifying alternative activities such as educational interests, employment opportunities, training opportunities, religious support groups, and recreational and cultural activities.

A children's group could be developed for the purposes of increasing awareness of American Indian customs and values and enhancing identification with American Indians. Objectives could be developed to (1) enhance the understanding of children's own tribal group and other tribal groups, (2) facilitate knowledge and awareness of current issues facing American Indian people today, (3) provide children opportunities to increase their skill level in American Indian activities, and (4) provide children with opportunities to discuss and positively enhance their own identification as an American Indian person.

Individual goals for members of an American Indian children's group could include the following: (1) developing American Indian beading abilities; (2) developing American Indian dancing abilities; (3) identifying other specific American Indian talents and developing these; (4) discussing one's American Indian heritage with a grandparent or other relative; (5) learning more about American Indian games and activities and teaching these to younger children; (6) developing awareness of American Indian cultural activities and participating in a program for school, family, or Indian gatherings; and (7) developing awareness of historical and current concerns of American Indian people and sharing this knowledge with others in school, at home, or with extended family members.

A task group may have the purpose of working to establish a halfway house for substance abusers. Objectives may include (1) provide support for one another in a group living situation, (2) provide education and information regarding aspects of problem drinking, (3) develop more successful problem solving skills, (4) develop interests in a variety of activities to more positively meet personal needs, and (5) provide group and individual counseling experiences to address the individual and group problems of the residents.

Social workers may find some client reluctance in setting goals or in planning particular activities or interventions to achieve goals. Some American Indian clientele come from tribal groups where they have been taught that to plan for or count on something in the future may actually deter its occurrence. It is important to address these issues in goal setting and planning activities, particularly where there is high interest of group participants, and tribal values and customs against pre-planning for such events.

Group rules should be utilized to facilitate group process and goal attainment. Rules should be negotiated with group members and should be kept at a minimum. Appropriate rules for groups may include (1) respect for each group member, (2) maintenance of confidentiality, (3) emphasis on courteous behavior—speaking for oneself and listening to others, (4) calling if unable to attend, (5) summarization of what has been learned at each session, and (6) discussion of how group members will implement such understanding outside the group.

Programming is most successful when a variety of activities and discussion topics are utilized. Indian films and filmstrips are particularly beneficial in spearheading discussion and promoting goal attainment. American Indian activities can be beneficial in enhancing attainment of cultural identification goals. Structured activities can promote specific goals such as problem solving and communication skill development. Structured activities enhance understanding and provide group members with opportunities to practice specific skills within the group setting. Many American Indians are open to participate in a variety of Indian and non-Indian activities. Older American Indian people have been motivated by participation in both indoor and outdoor activities including table games, charades, golf, bowling, and excursions. Group excursions to American Indian powwows and contests as well as recreational resorts are appealing to younger and older group members. It is important that programming enhance group members' attainment of individual goals and group purposes.

Termination of American Indian groups deserves important consideration. With some American Indian clientele it is difficult to express feelings of satisfaction or appreciation. It is the perception of many American Indian clients that the worker, being a bright and capable person, should understand the extent of the meaning of the group experience. Verbal expressions of appreciation and regard may, therefore, be given sparingly. However, the importance of the group experience should not be underestimated. It is not at all uncommon for social workers with little experience in working with American Indians to overestimate the depth of the professional relationship in the early stages of group intervention and to underestimate the importance of the professional relationship in the terminating phase of a group. It is recommended that attention be given to the termination process over a period of several weeks in preparing American Indian clients for a successful termination from a positive group experience.

TYPES OF GROUPS WHICH CAN BE FACILITATIVE
IN WORK WITH AMERICAN INDIAN CLIENTELE

Many group experiences have been successfully programmed for children, young adults, and older American Indian people. Boarding school groups have provided American Indian youth with opportunities to learn more about themselves, participate in worthwhile activities, deal with their individual and collective problems, and address future issues. Many American Indian youth attend boarding schools because they want to be educated within a system which serves other American Indians. They are also interested in learning more about their own culture and about the values and customs of other tribal groups. Group experiences in boarding schools could be programmed to help young people develop greater appreciation for their own culture, the cultures of other American Indian people, and an identification with Indians in general and with their own tribal group. At the beginning of a school year, American Indian youth could participate in a group experience which helps them identify the kinds of educational and personal experiences they would like to enjoy during the year. Activities could be programmed to facilitate their adjustment at the school and progress toward the achievement of these goals. All-Indian clubs could teach American Indian dances and songs. Individual interests and talents could be developed in art clubs, music clubs, outdoor clubs, and rodeo clubs. Personal development could be enhanced through attainment of communication or problem solving skills. Groups could be planned to provide education and prevention foci for dealing with topics such as drug and alcohol abuse. Therapy groups may offer treatment for people with drug and alcohol problems. Other therapy groups could address the social, behavioral, and personal problems of American Indian youth.

One boarding school has programmed a "New Beginnings" group experience. These groups address the needs of youth who have not made a satisfactory educational or behavioral adjustment to the boarding school. The "New Beginnings" focus is directed toward helping students learn more appropriate behaviors which retard their participation in anti-social or anti-educational activities, while providing rewards for positive behavior which allow them to remain in the educational setting. Other group experiences may deal with planning for the future. Young people could discuss experiences they could have in the armed services, at institutions of higher education, in technical/vocational schools, or with employment opportunities. Another group experience may be programmed to address tribal government issues and needs. These groups may stimulate young people to think about careers in tribal service, thus promoting the self-determination directions of tribal governments today.

Much attention has been given to the problems related to substance abuse among American Indian people. Groups are often facilitative in recovery house programs and in half-way houses. Out-reach programs from such settings could provide treatment for American Indian people with problem drinking behaviors who are otherwise functioning adequately within society. Prevention efforts could be addressed at the elementary school level and certainly at the junior and senior high levels. Work with families and the establishment of ALA-NON and ALA-TEEN groups within reservation and urban settings could also be beneficial.

Leadership groups could provide opportunities for leadership experiences appropriate for children, adolescents and adults. These group experiences could focus upon identification of leadership skills and provision of tangible experiences, wherein American Indian people could experience the satisfactions and frustrations of leadership assignments.

Educational groups could be beneficial to American Indian people at many levels. Assertiveness training group experiences may be particularly beneficial for adolescents, young adults in college settings, and adults in employment or leadership positions. Graduate students at institutions of higher education may find support groups helpful to them in learning about higher education systems and in providing encouragement and support to motivate continuation in graduate study programs. Adult education programs could provide opportunities for American Indian people to continue to learn, grow and develop personally, and to fill their time with rewarding and growth producing experiences.

Many youth groups could focus upon development of social skills and other skills as appropriate to meet their developmental needs. A particularly rewarding experience could be provided for young people to increase their cultural awareness and identification with American Indian people. Edwards et al. (1978) conducted such a group experience with American Indian girls at the University of Utah. This experience proved to be rewarding for the young women who participated in the group and for all members of their families who participated in some of their group activities and shared reports of the group experiences.

Women's groups and men's groups could address a variety of issues related to the needs and interests of American Indian men and women today. One such group might relate to the topic of roles of American Indian men and women—their current status, changes, and fluctuations. Parenting groups could address topics related to growth and development of children, pressures of parents in today's society, problems of single parents and blended families, and helping children achieve success. Other parenting groups may wish to discuss topics such as developing feelings of cultural and tribal identification among their children. Another group may wish to discuss the implications of inter-tribal marriages or mixed marriages (American Indian/non-Indian) upon themselves, their children, and their families.

Groups can provide interesting and rewarding experiences for American Indian elderly. Older American Indian people, (or so it seems to these authors) often develop a sereneness about them which frees their participation in many and varied group activities. There is often a blending felt in older American Indian groups. The laughter and displays of humor are contagious. Their willingness to try new experiences and to invest themselves in diversified activities can lead to many enjoyable group meetings. While it may be necessary to modify group activities because of aging, members highly value their participation. The sharing of food and activities contribute to a positive atmosphere. Group work with older American Indian people can be a most satisfying and refreshing experience for the older American Indian person and the social workers as well.

The use of task groups can be helpful in addressing the needs of American Indians. A task group could be formed to address the problem of housing among the aged or substance abusers or the handicapped. The establishment of therapeutic half-way houses could be facilitated through the efforts of American Indian task groups.

Other concerns which could be appropriate assignments for task groups include issues related to unemployment and stimulating industry or business ventures on reservations. American Indian tribal groups may wish to cooperate with one another in the establishment of educational programs, employment opportunities, housing for correctional purposes or for the handicapped, and the establishment of foster homes or group homes to meet child welfare needs. Other cooperative activities could facilitate programming of cultural events or social activities.

A task group could address the economic needs of American Indians, such as development of negotiating skills to deal with issues including the use and development of energy resources, water rights, trust funds, and leasing. Business administration principles could be helpful in analyzing appropriate business and hiring practices, such as implications of employing family and friends.

Another task group may wish to address issues related to providing appropriate models for Indian young people. Older American Indian people may become more actively involved with youth in an effort to promote more effective modeling. Adolescents may be similarly involved in modeling appropriate behavior for younger Indian children.

Some Indian tribal groups may wish to establish a task group to evaluate the needs of younger Indian children. Programs such as Head Start could promote training programs for children and parents. Community programs could be developed for pre-school experiences for young children.

Groups could be formed in urban settings to assist American Indians in making adjustments to new living situations. These groups could focus on helping Indian people deal with feelings of loss of satisfying associations they have, heretofore, experienced with extended families. Such groups may facilitate ''adoption'' of uncles, aunts, and grandparents in urban settings. Other American Indian people may appreciate group experiences which help them achieve a better adjustment to their employment situation and learn more about employment benefits such as medical insurance, day care, and sick leave. Another aspect of such a group may emphasize helping American Indians become better acquainted with community resources and become better integrated in the community, taking advantage of Indian and non-Indian resources. Such groups could also identify American Indian people who would be willing to serve on boards of American Indian programs in urban settings.

Children, adolescents, and adults could be encouraged to participate in groups which emphasize development of cultural skills and understanding of their own tribal customs and the values and customs of other tribal groups. Group members might be invited to make presentations to schools and community groups at times of

special events—Thanksgiving and Indian cultural or social gatherings—or the dedication of Indian edifices such as tribal buildings or
business enterprises.

Group work practice with American Indians can be a most satisfying and rewarding experience for both the American Indian
clientele and the social group worker. Programming possibilities are
unlimited. Personal growth and development of group members can
be greatly enhanced as members participate in well planned and
worth while group experiences. Such learning can be solidified
when group members are encouraged to practice new behaviors in
appropriate social situations outside the group.

SUMMARY

American Indians have traditionally enjoyed participation in a
variety of group experiences. Social workers can capitalize on these
cultural precedents and the current interest of many American Indian people in participating in groups. It is important to recognize
the uniqueness of each American Indian person and tribal group in
planning for social work intervention. Attempts at recognizing and
relating to such uniqueness are appreciated by American Indian people and facilitate social work intervention.

American Indian people are currently addressing many important
concerns. Recognition of such issues can provide the basis for social
group work intervention. Current concerns of both an individual
and tribal nature could be addressed within the group context. Social
group work planning could provide for individual problem solving,
tribal and community planning, and treatment and prevention possibilities.

Many American Indian people prefer to work with Native
American social workers. However, non-Indian social workers who
are sensitive to American Indian people have enjoyed considerable
success in their social work intervention with Native Americans. It
is important to understand the values of each individual Indian client
and tribal group with whom social workers practice.

Considerable attention should be directed toward establishment of
appropriate group purposes and individual goals and objectives.
Structuring the group for goal attainment is also an important consideration as is utilizing programming which directly relates to
group purposes and objectives. Termination is a crucial variable
which impacts upon the entire group experience.

The variety of group possibilities is as extensive as the creativity of the social group worker and the American Indian clientele being served. A variety of activities and discussions are recommended. Innovative and creative planning are encouraged. The successful implementation of social group work experiences with American Indian people can provide much satisfaction for the clientele they are designed to serve and the social workers who lead them.

REFERENCES

The American Indian family: Strengths and stresses. Proceedings of Conference on Research Issues. Phoenix, Arizona, April 17-19, 1980.

Edwards, E. D., Edwards, M. E., Daines, G. M., & Eddy, F. Enhancing self-concept and identification with "Indianness" of American Indian girls. *Social Work with Groups*, 1978, *1*(3), 309-318.

Hirsfelder, A. B. *American Indian stereotypes in the world of children: A reader and bibliography.* Metuchen, N. J.: Scarecrow Press, 1982.

Thornton, R., Sandefur, G. D., & Grasmick, H. G. *The urbanization of American Indians.* Bloomington: Indiana University Press, 1982.

Youngman, G., & Sadongei, M. Counseling the American Indian child. In D. R. Atkinson, G. Morten, & D. W. Sue (ed.), *Counseling American minorities: A cross-cultural perspective.* Dubuque, Iowa: Wm. C. Brown, 1979.

CALL FOR PAPERS

in conjunction with

THE CENTENNIAL CELEBRATION

of the

LIFE AND WORKS OF
BERTHA CAPEN REYNOLDS
1885-1978

PROGRAMS: AMERICAN ORTHOPSYCHIATRIC ASSOCIATION ANNUAL MEETING
New York City—Monday, April 22, 1985

SMITH COLLEGE SCHOOL FOR SOCIAL WORK
Northampton, MA—Weekend June 28-30, 1985

AWARDS: Up to six papers will be chosen to receive the Frank C. Bancroft Award ($500). Selected papers may be published.

CATEGORIES: Manuscripts from faculty, students and practitioners will be judged separately.

CRITERIA: Papers may deal with any aspect of Bertha C. Reynolds work and writing—her philosophy, teaching practice, relation to the labor movement, contributions to social policy, minority and women's issues, social work theory and social action. Examination of both the historical and contemporary relevance of Reynold's contributions is involved. Manuscripts will be judged on the basis of scholarship, creativity, contributions to the field and relevance to centennial purpose.

FORMAT: Manuscripts of up to 20 double spaced typewritten pages may be submitted (4 copies). Use of style guide recommended—Publication Manual of the American Psychological Association, 2nd edition, 1974.

DEADLINE: December 1, 1984. Submit manuscripts to *Dr. Catherine Riessman, Smith College School of Social Work, Northampton, MA 01063.* Selections announced March 16, 1985.

SELECTION COMMITTEE: Dr. George Getzel, Hunter College School of Social Work, Dr. Shirley Jenkins, Columbia University School of Social Work, Prof. Barbara Joseph, Hofstra University, Labor Studies Program, Dr. Catherine Riessman, Smith College School of Social Work.

Asian/Pacific-Americans
and Group Practice

Judy Chu
Stanley Sue

ABSTRACT. Although Asian/Pacific-Americans encounter a multitude of life stressors and have significant mental health needs, many avoid the use of psychotherapeutic services. This article argues that group practice can be efficacious in addressing their mental health needs if therapists appreciate and understand the cultural factors and historical background of these clients. Cultural and historical considerations are discussed within the context of the strategies (e.g., group content and structure, composition, and dynamics) to use.

The constant search for ethnically sensitive forms of psychotherapeutic treatment is especially crucial for Asian/Pacific-Americans. For this group, treatment within the traditional mental health system is new for users and practitioners alike, and the need for effective methods is painfully apparent. This article describes issues for Asian/Pacific-Americans in one form of psychotherapy—group treatment. The cultural and historical issues involved are discussed, and then specific recommendations are made for group practice.

In describing the Asian/Pacific-American population, it is important to be cautious about making generalizations. It is a population comprised of many different ethnic groups with diverse cultures and experiences. Certain Asian groups, such as the Chinese, Japanese, Korean, and Vietnamese have some differences in background from Pacific Islander groups such as Guamanians, Samoans, and Hawai-

Judy Chu is Lecturer in Asian-American Studies, University of California, Los Angeles. Stanley Sue is Professor of Psychology, University of California, Los Angeles.

23

ians. There are as many as 35 distinct Asian ethnic groups, each with cultural distinctions.

In addition to the ethnic uniqueness of each group, there are also differences in the immigration pattern of Asian/Pacific-Americans. Recent waves of immigrants from Korea, the Philippines, and Hong Kong are different from the refugees of Southeast Asia. Both these groups can then be distinguished from the third or fourth generation American-born Asian. There are varying degrees of influence that Asian cultural norms have had in the succeeding generations of Asian/Pacific-Americans. For these reasons, as much specific attention are paid to these distinctions as possible. Finally, in our discussion we attempt to indicate what Asian/Pacific clients may be experiencing. Our attempt in this discussion is to contrast Asian/Pacific and Western values and experiences rather than to stereotype one group or another.

CULTURAL FACTORS

When the Resthaven Community Mental Health Center existed in the early 1970s on the edge of Los Angeles' Chinatown, residents would walk on the other side of the street because they did not want to be associated with that "crazy house." Asian/Pacific-American immigrants frequently view those who are mentally ill with rejection and ridicule, and hesitate to admit the existence of such persons within their family (Chien and Yamamoto, 1982). Such attitudes are reflected in the consistent under-utilization rates of Asian/Pacific-Americans in the mental health care system (Hatanaka, Watanabe, and Ono, 1975; Sue and McKinney, 1980). There are many factors giving rise to Asian under-utilization. First, mental health services have had difficulty adapting to the cultures and languages of Asian/Pacific-American communities. Secondly, there are cultural values inhibiting utilization, such as the feeling that taking care of one's personal problems indicates greater maturity, or that one should not reveal intimate details to strangers (Murase, 1979). The western concept of "paying to talk" has not been accepted by a significant proportion of the community.

However, as Asians assimilate into America, cultural traditions and stability break down. Some Asians live in ethnic enclaves like Chinatown, Manilatown, and Little Tokyo, but many do not and therefore face the pressures of assimilation. Socio-economic pressures make survival a great challenge. Cultural continuity from generation to generation is difficult. In this new context, mental health workers are needed to help Asian/Pacific-Americans through the inevitable adjustment process.

The cultural differences between Asians and Americans in the area of mental health have been well documented (Clement, 1974; Shon, 1979; Sue and Morishima, 1982; Sue and Sue, 1979; Yamamoto, 1978). Of course, such cultural norms are strongest for those who have recently arrived and varies in strength with succeeding generations. It is important to note, however, that the Asian/Pacific-American population is a relatively new grouping in America with many spanning, at the most, three generations.

Asian/Pacifics bring to America some norms that directly contradict with those of western psychological thought. Western psychotherapy emphasizes independence and self-sufficiency. Individual life achievement and self-growth are considered important. Maturity is marked by independence from the family. Asian/Pacific Americans emphasize interdependence and collectivity. Tasks are taken and plans made with the family in mind. "Filial piety" is a powerful concept in which obligations to parents must be respected throughout life. Family roles tend to be highly structured.

Such respect is maintained throughout life by means of the indirect control of parents. Asian/Pacific-American children are not trained to respond to direct punishment, but are socialized according to methods using guilt and shame. For example, the worst punishment given a young Asian female child could be that tasks be taken from her, therefore proving her incompetence (Fillmore and Cheong, 1980). Asian parents scold children by referring to how the children's behavior reflects on the family (Ho, 1976). Given lifelong training in indirect communication, the western psychotherapeutic method of direct confrontation and criticism is often an affront to Asian/Pacific-American sensibilities.

In western psychotherapy, the expression of feelings is frequently considered therapeutic or of therapeutic value. The verbalization of such feelings is an indication of greater self-growth and perhaps the abandonment of repressed or suppressed experiences. In Asian cultures, the expression of feelings has a utilitarian purpose as well. One example is the extraordinary effort it took for first generation Asians to survive in America. Many harsh conditions were faced with a sense of stoicism in which feelings of self-pity or defeat were subdued for the overall good. Contemporary examples are found in

Indochinese refugees who face enormous cultural and socioeconomic changes in their abrupt move to the United States, but find it important as a strategy for survival to show that they can endure (Tung, 1980).

Attitudes toward authority are different. In western psychotherapy, the therapist oftentimes has an ambiguous role, sometimes being friend and sometimes advisor. Asians expect a more formal relationship, especially since they have gone to the extraordinary measure of coming to a therapist. They are expecting expertise and competence, and a somewhat more formal relationship with the therapist. Nakao and Lum (1977) did, indeed, find that Asian-American professionals tended to be more formal in their treatment of Asian-American clients. Many Asians do not want to have to solve the problem themselves, but expect the therapist to take an active role in therapy.

In western psychotherapy, the concept of the unconscious has had a great deal of influence. Many actions are seen as the product of hidden motivation. Thus, illnesses can be seen as part of a more profound problem. Many Asians do come into psychotherapy with psychophysiological complaints, which may, indeed, reflect more underlying problems. However, rather than detracting from the solution to the problem, the client sees the illness as part of the totality of the problem.

In feudal Asian cultures, women take a secondary role to men (Homma-True, 1980). The long history of Confucianism has pervaded the hierarchical thinking of many Asian/Pacific-Americans. As immigrants come to the United States, they find that much different norms exist. However, some are not able to adjust so quickly. Thus, one must be aware of male/female dynamics. An Asian woman immigrant may feel very uncomfortable being alone with a male therapist and telling him her intimate secrets. This may also be true for male clients/female therapists.

HISTORICAL FACTORS

The societal experience of being Asian in America is an integral factor in treating Asian/Pacific-Americans (Kitano and Matsushima, 1976). Asian/Pacific-Americans have had a long history of discrimination, ranging from the anti-immigration laws of 1882 to the concentration camps of World War II and to the more recent resentment against "boat people." An inconsistent contrast to these blatantly negative stereotypes is another image that has arisen within the last decade, that of the "model minority." Sex-roled stereotypes face similar inconsistency. Asian women have been given stereotypes that range from exotic and dangerous to passive and subservient. Asian men were seen historically as menaces to white women but many now complain of being seen as "emasculated." Such wide inconsistencies in Asian/Pacific-American images have frequently generated ambivalent feelings of Asians toward their own race and toward the mainstream society.

In some cases, the effect of discrimination has had obvious psychological effects. One example is that of the concentration camps. The recent hearings held across the United States have shown that much more trauma was experienced than was at first admitted by Japanese-Americans (Commission on Wartime Relocation, 1981). While the effects varied by generation and sex, Mass (1978) found that Japanese-Americans felt betrayed by a trusted source. Niseis had especially been loyal Americans, and were numbed when they found that they had been scapegoated. They suppressed such feelings because the reality was too painful to face.

While such societally-based psychological problems are too many to delve into in this article, they are important enough for the therapist to investigate further. However, common problems that may arise in a group setting include image problems, generational conflicts, and relationship problems.

Regarding image problems, both immigrant and American-born Asians must cope with the negative or stereotypic images American society has of them. Immigrants must cope with the changing norms in American society and the sometimes negative views with which those who do not speak English well are viewed. American-born Asians oftentimes have identity problems since they do not have many models with which to follow.

Generational conflicts occur when children assimilate faster than parents, yet parents pressure children to maintain the old culture. Children, knowing the English language and western culture better than parents, sometimes operate as a semiauthority figure, changing the dynamics of the family relationship. They may become ashamed of their parents' ways.

Regarding relationship problems, Asian women and men oftentimes have negative views of one another as romantic partners due to their adherence to American beauty standards and personality norms. Interracial relationships are becoming common, but they also engender problems because of the reactions of family and society.

GROUP STRATEGIES

Nakao and Lum (1977) report that Asian-American psychotherapists prefer to see their clients in individual psychotherapy. Some feel that the individual approach would be more appropriate than the group approach because it is less threatening to the Asian/Pacific-American, who has enough reluctance to talk about such problems to one stranger, let alone several.

Group work, however, may prove quite beneficial in ways that individual psychotherapy cannot. The Asian/Pacific client who values interdependence and cooperation can gain much from the power and strength of collective group feedback. In a group of Asian-Americans, members can be very supportive of one another in patterns already familiar to the Asian-American client. Like family members, they will work together to solve one member's problems. If the Asian-American is in a group of non-Asians, the Asian can find much benefit in learning about others' communication styles. Modeling can teach the Asian how to be assertive or how to express feelings. Seeing other lifestyles can teach an Asian/Pacific-American the flexibility offered by different norms, therefore providing more ways of solving a problem.

In some ways, the group atmosphere can be less threatening than individual psychotherapy. Rather than being constantly pressured to talk, as in individual psychotherapy, the Asian/Pacific-American in group sessions can choose when to interact. In individual psychotherapy, the pressure of attention given to the client may be an inhibiting factor, in and of itself. It typically is a more one-sided relationship in which the therapist does the giving and the client the receiving. In the group setting, the Asian is not only the recipient, but the helper. The sense of obligation that an Asian could feel would be ameliorated. Furthermore, some of the socially-oriented problems that Asians have, such as self-image or assertion problems, can be worked on right in the group. The client can try alternate behaviors and therefore see that the problem is workable.

However, the problems that Asians face in group practice are obvious. Asians may feel more inhibited in talking and in expressing deep feelings. Feelings of shame about failures in life may have difficulty being brought to light. In family work, Asian/Pacific-Americans may be reluctant to talk about members of the family in front of them. Children do not want to be disrespectful to parents, and parents are cautious about revealing intimate details about themselves in front of children (McDermott, Tseng, and Maretzki, 1980). The Asian client may not want to talk about family members in ways that imply disrespect. Asians in mixed groups may feel inhibited. If the rest of the group is very talkative and assertive, the Asian/Pacific-American may be at disadvantage. The Asian may feel it is impolite to interrupt others, or that it is the height of narcissism and egomania to "monopolize" a session with their problem. Because of these possible problems, the therapist must think of different strategies more appropriate to the Asian/Pacific-American.

Content and Structure of Group

The therapist must balance size and content of group if appealing to the Asian/Pacific-American clients. If the group has a fairly structured content, such as in an assertiveness training program, the group can be fairly large. The largeness of the group may, in fact, serve the purpose of allowing the Asian to feel safer, since so many others see such an activity as valuable. Structured content may also help in making the Asian feel comfortable with the purpose of the group. Structured-content groups would have Asian-specific themes. For instance, groups in balancing family and career, on succeeding in America, or on assertiveness training may lead to deeper problem-solving, yet be safe enough to at least try.

The deeper the group gets into content, however, the more group size will be an inhibitor. A larger group should break down into smaller components; a small size of seven or eight people may be more appropriate.

The Asian community is so diverse that groups with people of common background would work best together. For instance, convening a group of war brides may be the only way to reach such a population. The younger generation, especially teenage youth, will have problems and communication styles much different from their parents' generation.

Ho (1976) suggests that in family therapy such differences are so great that different mental health workers are needed to target the different members of the family. Thus, he cites the case study of parents and a troubled child in which a different worker was needed for the wife, the husband, and the child.

Composition of Group

There are varied advantages and disadvantages to consider in mixing Asians in an ethnically diverse group as opposed to keeping them in one that is homogeneously Asian.

The greatest problem in mixed groups is that the style of verbal communication that Asians have is often different from others. Asians tend not to interrupt another or push to make their point. Asians may take longer to answer a question. In a group of very verbose, articulate, and aggressive non-Asians, the Asian member may be hesitant to speak up. In a confrontation, which inevitably happens at some point in a long-term group, the Asian may not know what to say, not being used to such interaction.

Sometimes, the Asian client is ready to assert him/herself into a group and wants to model after other people's styles. But in the initial stages in which an Asian is first considering a group, it may be more beneficial for Asians to be placed within a group of other Asian/Pacific-Americans, especially when dealing with sensitive problems. Such a group can sense one another's communication and may thus be more empathetic. Equal participation by Asians would also facilitate the development of leadership skills of some members within the group. Unfortunately, in a mixed group, Asians may not take the lead in intervening in another's problems. They may reinforce their view of themselves as followers rather than leaders or helpers.

Group Dynamics

The Asian/Pacific-American frequently expects the therapist to fulfill his/her role as the director of activity in group. Thus, Tung (1980) writes that most Asian/Pacific clients wait for active probing by the therapist or an expressed invitation to speak. The therapist needs to be directive at first to set the tone for the Asian in the group. This needs to be done in a non-threatening, non-confrontive manner. The therapist, in his/her own role as the director, suggests that a change in behavioral interaction are permitted and safe—and perhaps necessary in order to solve problems. Calling on group members to talk shows that it is permitted; knowing when to stop lets them know its safe.

The therapist can facilitate this process of verbalizing feelings by interpreting nonverbal communication into verbal communication. Because a person is not talking does not mean that the person is not paying attention. A group member may in fact be paying avid attention to the group, but may be censoring his/her own input. Watching for subtle changes in nonverbal communication is crucial to understanding the dynamics of the Asian group. Care and concern for the group may be expressed through deeds, not words. For instance, in Asian groups, members inevitably bring food to convey closeness. In one case, a member always took pictures of the members of the group and passed them out. Such deeds are important to recognize and reinterpret verbally.

The emphasis on collectivity of Asians means that they may be reluctant to express any doubts or criticisms of the group. The group worker would benefit by anticipating them and bringing them to the surface. Allowing doubts to be expressed is an important part of confidence-building and leadership training. Ho (1976) describes an interaction in which the many silences of an Asian-American group was broken when one group member ventured forth to talk about how such silences bothered him. The interaction was an important turning point for the group.

The degree of physical contact in Asian cultures is very different from that which exists in other cultures. Physical contact is not taken as casually as it is in mainstream America, especially heterosexual contact. Humanistic modes of psychotherapy may find physical contact integral to closeness, but among Asians lines of distinction are drawn between private and public shows of physical affection. The psychotherapist must be conscious of when and with whom to have such contact, especially in regard to the opposite sex.

Reassessing Values

Given the different historical/cultural conditions from which Asian/Pacific-Americans came, the goals of group psychotherapy can be redefined in order to make them culturally specific. There are clearly identifiable value changes that can be made that would help an Asian/Pacific-American to function more effectively in the American society.

Self-esteem. The Asian/Pacific cultures do not emphasize one's own development, but one's development in relationship to and in cooperation with others. This value may be maintained at the expense of one's own self-definition and self-esteem. In fact, the Asian/Pacific-American may even think it selfish to think of him/herself. Added to this are stereotyped media images and discrimination. With that, and the lack of positive role models in key leadership positions in American society, Asian/Pacific-Americans would have to be quite resourceful to come up with positive images for themselves. An Asian-American, not aware of such obstacles, may internalize many problems. The group process can serve to separate the problems borne by outer society as opposed to those with origins in the inner self (intra psychic).

It is obvious that the Asian needs validation of the self. The group can provide that validation. It can give direct feedback as to that person's strengths, and can give permission for one to think of one's strengths.

The following example illustrates how important such validation is:

> A young Filipino-American male responded spontaneously in group to another's statement, and some members laughed, though not maliciously. However, he was quiet for a couple of sessions afterwards. Outside of group, he asked the therapist whether he should say things in the group, because he felt stupid that time that he did. The therapist encouraged him to continue to speak, and reinterpreted the event. He did start to speak again, and eventually shared much about himself in the group.

Assertion of feelings. The Asian cultural value of privacy or inconspicuousness may be appropriate in Asia; but in America, verbal assertiveness may make the difference in a promotion, in success in a job interview, or between an A or a B grade in school. Confidence in speaking is perhaps one factor in explaining why Asians are not in upper-management jobs nor in high visibility jobs (Cabezas, 1979).

Similarly, interpersonal relationships are much more ambiguous in American than they are in Asia. Interpersonal roles in marriage and family are much more defined in Asian countries. But in America, there is much more active personal interaction that is required in all roles such as in seeking and courting a mate, in soliciting cooperation from fellow workers, and in dealing with family relations. Interestingly, a recent study (Yeung, 1982) showed that interracial Chinese-American couples tended to adjust better to one another because the differences in their cultures forced them to assert their feelings and examine their differences. In contrast, the Chinese-Chinese couples tended to assume similarities in their relationships. Thus, asserting one's feelings is possible and helpful to the survival of the Asian/Pacific-American.

The lack of permission to assert feelings sometimes results in feeling out of control when one does reveal oneself.

A young Japanese-American woman oftentimes looked as though she were about to say something in the group. She would be encouraged by others to talk in the group, and slowly she eventually did open up. When she did talk about herself, her family, or boyfriend, tears would often well up and she would become inarticulate. Her awareness of her tears often immobilized her from expressing herself as freely as she liked.

Asserting one's feelings can simply be posed as a reorientation in philosophy, and thus can be stressed in a non-threatening manner. Such expression can be functional, preventing illness and helping one to perform more freely in everyday functions. Knowing oneself can help the client in everyday cooperation and interaction.

Role-playing particular situations that are feeling-laden can serve to separate the client from the problem, can involve the group, and can concretize the problem.

Understanding family and community. Ambivalence toward one's heritage and family upbringing is fairly common among Asian/Pacific-Americans. Some undergo tremendous amounts of pressures to fulfill family expectations whereas others are rebellious against family standards. Ambivalence toward the family is partly imposed by the pressure to assimilate according to American standards. Yet, the Asian cannot turn his/her back on the culture. Setting boundaries and clarifying expectations is very important for the Asian/Pacific American who must cope with two cultures whose standards are strongly expressed. Members of a group can play an important role in supportively challenging the member's expectations.

A middle-aged Chinese-American male felt pressure to be a responsible son, but resented his parents for being continuously critical of him. They wanted to live with him, but he didn't want them to and was ashamed of his thoughts. The group, all Asian, talked about their own experiences with their parents. The client eventually acknowledged his different feelings and bought them a house nearby his own.

CONCLUSION

There are many and varied sources of stress in being an Asian/ Pacific person in America. Potential problems range from the culture shock experienced by the immigrant to the conflicts of identity, discrimination, and/or interracial marriage faced by the American-born. Psychotherapy can be quite beneficial in facilitating the process of working through these dilemmas appropriately.

To be effective, the psychotherapeutic approach must be sensitive to the cultural values of the Asian/Pacific-American while at the same time be careful not to stereotype this richly diverse group of people. It is clear that some of the premises upon which traditional western psychotherapeutic methods are built clash directly with Asian cultural values. The social worker must be aware of an Asian emphasis on obligation to the family, respecting authority, valuing group needs over the individual, and not "showing off."

Such values have led some to believe that group practice would be too inhibiting for Asian/Pacific-American clients. For the Asian/ Pacific who has a stigma attached to sharing problems publicly, a group certainly could reinforce any reluctance to express deep feelings of self-doubt or guilt. However, group work can be used quite beneficially if viewed from a different perspective. Given the emphasis in Asian cultures on collectivity, feedback from many can have far more impact than individual interaction. Moreover, Asians can develop the social skills that are necessary for survival in American society.

In order to be successful, some factors must be taken into consideration in utilizing the group method. A mixed ethnic group may inhibit Asian input due to the different verbal communication styles. The male/female composition must be considered due to the hierarchical sex roles in Asian society. A more structured approach may be helpful in teaching the Asian/Pacific client how to be in such a group.

The group can especially be helpful in reassessing values. Thus, through feedback from others, one may gain self-esteem and confidence. Through the practice of expressing feelings, the Asian/ Pacific-American may become more assertive. Finally, through the shared experiences of other Asian/Pacific-Americans, the client may gain a larger perspective with which to understand the cultural pressures inherent in the Asian/Pacific family and community.

REFERENCES

Cabezas, A. Disadvantages employment status of Asian- and Pacific-Americans. In the U.S. Commission Civil Rights, *Civil rights issues of Asian- and Pacific-Americans.* Washington D.C.: U.S. Government Printing Office, 1979.

Chien, C.P., & Yamamoto, J. Asian-Americans and Pacific Islander patients. In F.X. Acosta, J. Yamamoto and L.A. Evans (Eds.) *Effective psychotherapy for low-income and minority patients.* New York: Plenum Press, 1982.

Clement, D.C. *Samoan concepts of mental illness and treatment.* Unpublished doctoral dissertation, University of California, Irvine, 1974.

Commission on Wartime Relocation and Internment of Civilians. Selected testimonies from the Los Angeles and San Francisco hearings. *Amerasia Journal,* 1981, *8,* 55-105.

Fillmore, L.W., & Cheong, J.C. The early socialization of Asian-American female children. In National Institute of Education, *Conference on the educational and occupational needs of Asian/Pacific-American women.* Washington D.C.: U.S. Government Printing Office, 1980.

Hatanaka, H., Watanabe, B., & Ono, S. The utilization of mental health services in the Los Angeles area. In W. Ishikawa, and N. Archer (Eds.), *Service delivery in Pan-Asian communities.* San Diego: Pacific/Asian Coalition, 1975.

Ho, M.K. Social work with Asian-Americans. *Social Casework,* 1976, *57,* 195-201.

Homma-True, R. Mental health issues among Asian-American women. In National Institute of Education, *Conference on the educational and occupational needs of Asian/Pacific-American women.* Washington D.C.: U.S. Government Printing Office, 1980.

Kitano, H.H.L., & Matsushima, N. Counseling Asian-Americans. In P.P. Pedersen, J.G. Draguns, W.J. Conner, & J.E. Trimble (Eds.), *Counseling across cultures.* Honolulu: University Press of Hawaii, 1981.

Mass, A.I. Socio-psychological effects of the concentration camp experience on Japanese-Americans. *Bridge: An Asian-American Perspective,* 1978, *6,* 61-63.

McDermott, J.F., Tsent, W.S. and Maretzki, T.W. (Eds.). *People and cultures of Hawaii: A psychocultural profile.* Honolulu: University Press of Hawaii, 1980.

Murase, K. State and local public policy issues in delivering mental health and related services to Asian- and Pacific-Americans. In U.S. Commission on Civil Rights, *Civil rights issues of Asian- and Pacific-Americans.* Washington D.C.: U.S. Government Printing Office, 1979.

Nakao, S., & Lum, C. *Yellow is not white and white is not right: Counseling techniques for Japanese and Chinese clients.* Unpublished masters thesis, University of California, Los Angeles, 1977.

Sue, D.W., & Sue, S. Counseling Chinese Americans. In D.R. Atkinson, G. Morten, & D.W. Sue, *Counseling American minorities: A cross-cultural perspective.* Dubuque, Iowa: Wm. C. Brown, 1979.

Sue, S., & McKinney, H. Asian-Americans in the community mental health care system. In R. Endo, S. Sue, and N.N. Wagner (Eds.), *Asian-Americans: social and psychological perspectives, volume II.* Palo Alto, Calif.: Science and Behavior Books, 1980.

Sue, S., & Morishima, J.K. *The mental health of Asian-Americans.* San Francisco: Jossey-Bass, 1982.

Tung, T.M. *Indochinese patients: Cultural aspects of the medical and psychiatric care of Indochinese refugees.* Washington D.C.: Action for Southeast Asians, Inc., 1980.

Yamamoto, J. Therapy for Asian-Americans. *Journal of the American Medical Association*, 1978, *70*, 267-270.

Yeung, W.T. *Chinese outmarriage in Los Angeles County.* Unpublished doctoral dissertation, University of California, Los Angeles, 1982.

Group Work Practice
with Asian Clients:
A Sociocultural Approach

Peter C. Lee
Gordon Juan
Art B. Hom

ABSTRACT. While considerable interest has been given to the social work with Asian-Americans, little attention has been paid to the Asian group work practice. This article suggests a sociocultural approach in working with Asian groups, including a knowledge of the sociocultural heritage of the Asian clients, the proper respect for the members of the family on group process, and the group worker's awareness of the significance of role expectation and its meaning for clients. In dealing with these sociocultural aspects, the social worker's role in Asian group treatment is that of a culture broker and enabler.

In the past decade the size and composition of Asian- and Pacific-Americans—now numbered more than 3.5 million—underwent a transformation of such a magnitude that their final configurations defy definition. Associated with these developments is a heightened awareness of the diversity of the Asian and Pacific Islander population and concerns over their special needs and problems. While the social work profession has shown considerable interest in Asian-Americans (Kitano, 1971; Kuramoto, 1971; Ozawa, 1972; Kim,

Peter C. Lee, MSW, MPH, DSW, is Associate Professor, School of Social Work, San Jose State University, Washington Square, San Jose, California 95192. Gordon Juan, MD, is Director of Clinical Services, Asian Community Mental Health Services, 310 8th Street, Oakland, California 94607. Art B. Hom, MSW, LCSW, is Director of Community Crisis Clinics, Mount Zion Hospital and Medical Center, 2415 Sutter Street, San Francisco, California 94115.

1973; Murase, 1973; Ho, 1976; Toupin, 1980; Montero and Dieppa, 1982), little attention has been given to the Asian group work practices. This article describes the aims, advantages, limitations, and ways in which social workers can provide culturally relevant group interventions. The emphasis is primarily on the sociocultural factors that are unique among Asian-Americans or that require special attention when such interventions are applied in Asian groups. For the purposes of this article, the term "Asian-American" refers to persons of Chinese, Japanese, Korean, Filipino, Pacific Islander, and Southeast Asian ancestry.

ASIAN CULTURES IN CONTEXT

Before discussing the sociocultural approach of group intervention for Asian clients, social group workers need to understand the current state of art and sociocultural factors underlying Asian cultures. A recurring theme in the literature related to Asian-Americans has to do with the appropriateness of current clinical social work approaches. While the literature has few empirical studies, the consensus is that Western treatment modalities based on nondirective techniques are inappropriate for ethnic minority groups (Sue and McKinney, 1975; Hong and Tsukashima, 1980; Morales, 1981). The irrelevance of social work interventions to Asians is frequently implied as a reason for their underutilization of human services (Matsushima and Tashima, 1982). Further, Asian clients are generally inclined to use health and welfare services that are culturally sensitive to their needs (Salicido, Nakano, and Jue, 1980). A commonly held assumption is that Western treatment modalities tend to minimize sociocultural factors in assessment, and, therefore, may affect the process of interpersonal interactions and communications between social workers and Asian clients.

For group intervention to be therapeutically effective, members are expected to share their problems and to express ideas and feelings openly. Such admission of problems in particular is perceived as a lack of self-control and will power; and as a family defect, open sharing of problems in a group situation is intolerable for most Asian-Americans (Ho, 1976). Free participation and exchange of views in treatment groups appears to be in conflict with Asian values of humility and modesty, as the following experience indicates.

Mr. V, a 23-year-old Vietnamese college student, was having an adjustment reaction with anxiety and depression from a psychiatric perspective, precipitated by his recent arrival in this country. Although Mr. V was active and had been the most verbal member of the group, he suddenly became very quiet during the group session. When asked by the worker for the reason of his silences, Mr. V revealed that he had heard of dissatisfactions among some members of the group regarding his "attention-seeking" and "show-off" behaviors. It is better to be quiet than to speak out so frequently. Those who do speak out frequently are not well thought of or appreciated, according to Mr. V.

The concept of obligation is also crucial. In American society, the tendency toward reciprocity is weighed heavily toward contractual obligation, agreed upon freely among group members. Within Asian cultures, obligation is important and is generally incurred through ascribed roles or status or through kindness or helpfulness received from other people. At times, obligations to different individuals may conflict and become a source of great anxiety (Shon and Ja, 1982).

In Asian cultures where interdependence is emphasized, the actual or perceived withdrawal of support may shake the individual's basic trust and confidence and raise one's anxiety of being alone. Thus, the fear of losing face can be a motivating force for one's conformity in group encounters. Because mutually respected interpersonal relationships are highly regarded in Asian groups, any direct or open confrontation which may lead to disagreement and loss of face for people involved is avoided whenever possible. Therefore, much of the communication style of Asian group tends to be indirect (Ho, 1976; Shon and Ja, 1982).

While the critics, such as Doi (1973), Sue and Sue (1973), and Yamamoto (1978) suggest that Asians often do not share Western values of independence (versus interdependence), individualism (versus familialism or groups), and assertiveness (versus indirectiveness), group work practice which is sensitive and conforms to Asian cultural values and family structure, however, can produce positive results (Chang, 1972; Ho, 1976). On the basis of this observation, we wish to share our knowledge and experience in the group treatments of dysfunctional Asian-Americans.

SOCIOCULTURAL APPROACH IN ASIAN GROUPS

Preparing for the Group Treatment

The process of entering group treatment is not an easy one for Asian-Americans. One of the most important principles to recognize in the pre-group screening of an Asian client for group therapy is that the successful engagement of that client into the group and the successful utilization of the group process for personal change is ultimately dependent upon the development of a trusting relationship between the client, the family, and the future group leader. The fact that the client's family must in some way be engaged in order for treatment to be successful is probably true of most forms of therapy with Asian clients, whether they are group-based or individually-based. The degree to which this pertains to a particular Asian client is related to the extent to which that client has continued to internalize his role within the family structure as a significant part of his identity. And the degree to which this is true depends in part on the extent of acculturation to Western sociocultural ideals versus those of a traditional culture. In the therapeutic group situation, the issue of exposure of personal or family "secrets" or "problems" into a relatively public setting is accentuated. The risk may be viewed as jeopardizing not just the individual involved, but the family as well. The future group worker must explicitly work toward becoming accepted by the family network as being a "member" versus "non-member" before effective group engagement will occur.

> Phi H. is a 8-year-old Cantonese-speaking Chinese boy referred to our Children's Clinic for temper tantrums and difficulty with peer relationships. The initial evaluation of child and family indicated a close, clinging relationship between mother and child with consequently exceedingly poor social skills development on the part of the child. Though the worker recognized that group therapy would be an important adjunct to treatment for the child quite early in the diagnostic/treatment process, he focused his attention on the development of a trusting relationship with the mother. Traditional sharing of the written symbols of their family names and identification of the worker's home province in China were important portions of this process. There were a number of collateral sessions with the mother before the issue of group treatment was intro-

duced and initiated. On the first day of his entry into the group, Phi H. was resistant, clinging to his mother and demonstrating significant separation anxiety. The mother gently entreated him to go and murmured to him, "It's okay, go with Uncle." With only mild further encouragement, Phi H. was able to join the group on his own.

If the group worker can become a trusted "member" of the family by both the client and his family, there is then the implicit understanding that the discussion of family or internal conflicts does not represent a public display and therefore does not incur a "loss of face" or humiliation. Nevertheless, the entry into the group therapy situation with its multiple strangers remains a threat. The worker is wise to meet with and seek explicit or implicit approval of the endeavor from the formal family leader (often the father or older male figure) or from the informal family leader (often the mother). This may necessitate several more sessions to meet with family members than would be usual in the evaluation and treatment of a non-Asian client. The sharing of personal information by the worker, though frowned upon by classically trained therapists, may be a necessary feature of the engagement process and should be understood as the equivalent of the Western handshake.

The Group Process

The process of unconscious identification of the therapeutic agent as being "part of the family" extends into the group process. For example:

> During the initial phase of a therapeutic group consisting of schizophrenic Asian men, considerable time was spent in recounting where each member had come from and what they had done during their lives. Each member shared different aspects of their personal history—some focused more on their education, others on their history of work, and still others on their "experience" or travels. All, however, made a point of where and when they were born. The rank ordering of the group largely followed the order of age seniority and "expertise." When seen individually, each had been distant and withdrawn and within the group there developed a cheerful comraderie. Eventually, under the urging of the workers, each

member agreed in turn to bring a snack for the group members to nibble on during their sessions.

The surprising level of familiarity and giving is attributable to the rapid acceptance at the unconscious level of the therapeutic group as a "family" versus "non-family" agent. Considerable attention is given to the rank order of each member within the group with maximal status attributed to the group leader and/or the worker. One can understand this process as a re-capitulation of dynamics from within the traditional extended Asian family. The transference to the group worker has been termed "messianic," though we prefer to understand it as "grandparental." The group worker is seen as having more knowledge, influence, and wisdom than even the parents who are somehow lacking and needing the assistance of the worker, as occurs often in the multigenerational extended Asian families, where the grandparents are asked to settle the more profound and weighty family problems. However, this grandparental transference by the individual Asian group member can have negative and positive effects. If allowed to remain unconscious, it can foster continued dependence on the group worker for solutions to personal or group problems with constriction of creative individual initiatives. The worker's counter-transference response may compel him or her to find solutions to difficult problems that might best be worked on by the group.

In addition, there is the risk of reinforcing the isolating, role-oriented hierarchical relationships so often found in Asian families, which, in turn, reduces the level of intimacy within the group. The group worker may be seduced by the excessively polite and considerate treatment he or she receives and lose sight of the costs of such treatment to the group. Nevertheless, such a position of power and unquestioned authority can be used consciously and constructively to provide much needed structure to more disturbed group members and to mobilize avoidant, anxious, or depressed clients. Given the nature of the unconscious transference, each positive reinforcement and each prohibition by the group worker carries enormous weight and impact. This can often reinforce a powerful prohibition within Asian groups (and within Asian families); the prohibition against violence, physical or verbal, is strong and monolithically hierarchical. That is to say that verbal or physical violence is only permissible when it occurs to a lower ranking group member. To even a greater extent than normally instilled by parental figures, the enormous weight of the authority given to the group worker often inhibit the verbal expression of hostility or physical violence between members of equal status or from lower to higher status members of the group.

The group worker should understand displays of aggression as possible displacements of anger downward, rather than the direct prohibited expression toward a higher status group member or group worker. Therefore, one's rank and status in the group is expected to place limits on the amount of and the direction of aggression or hostility within the Asian group. An Asian group member would expect minimal aggressive impulses directed from those below him or her in rank but might expect and accept aggressive behaviors from those above. To experience aggression from someone theoretically below oneself in the group hierarchy might signal a drop in that member's ranking within the social hierarchy of the group. Such an occurrence may raise concern and anxiety about the possible withdrawal of group support from its members. Likewise to experiencing confrontation or aggression beyond the level "permitted" or exceeding the normal range allowed within the group would raise similar concerns. Such open confrontation are therefore avoided in group or "public settings" and reserved for one-to-one confrontations, where concern over one's rank in the group is less likely to contaminate the issue. The Asian group members, because of their predominant transference to the group as being like an extended family, are, therefore, more likely to repress or suppress personal ID impulses in order to promote continued group harmony.

The issue of mixed-sex groups versus single-sex groups within Asian clients may best be discussed at this point. Hierarchical and social roles are reinforced on two fronts: the strict prohibition of incestuous fantasies (and the threat of acting them out) and the displacement of aggression to the lower status women or girls. The following case vignette demonstrates our point.

> Ken was a 10-year-old Asian youth who was seen in a mixed sex children's group. He was experiencing problems with significant impulsivity and inappropriate physical aggressiveness in school. Angry over his perceived lack of attention from the female group leader, he singled out the only white girl in the group and ranted and raved for several minutes about how he hated whites.

Aside from the issue of racial prejudice, this example illustrates the method of displacement and externalization (toward a white female) of aggression as well as the avoidance of sexual strivings toward the female Asian group leader and other Asian group members. As a consequence of the continued extensive identification with the family, one should expect to also see clearer evidence of sibling transferences among Asian group members, especially among peer group members.

The Group Ending Phase

The special meaning of the group termination must be understood by group workers so that they can be therapeutic, since a great deal is determined at this stage. Ideally, termination should occur when a group member or a total group no longer needs the professional services. The need for ending the group should be discussed well in advance of the expected termination date in order to allow group members sufficient time to make it a positive experience and to reduce hostility and anxiety among group members.

At this phase, a group worker should recapitalize on the knowledge and authority perceived and respected by the group members in making termination plans, including the follow-up services through individual counseling to group members if necessary. Therefore, the group worker must take a more direct stance toward the beneficial results of a "good" group termination experience. Thus, the worker may direct the group as to where each member and the group is in relation to group goals and to agency policies concerning the length of service and criteria for ending the group process.

In our view, the termination phase of group treatment is also strongly influenced by the "family" transference. There may be continued resistance to termination, and attempts at perpetuation of relationships between group members, as well as between group members and the worker beyond the ending date of the group. This continued dependence on "family relationships" points out two important sociocultural functions of the extended family to Asian clients. First, the family as an entity is included as a significant internalized object, introject, or part of the self. To separate would be to lose too large a portion of one's identity. Secondly, the family is also seen as a necessary link to immortality and is a defense against the various anxieties (separation, existential) so often verbalized in

Western culture. Contrary to Western ideas, the Asian client is more likely to see the family and, therefore, perhaps the therapeutic experience in groups as potentially helpful rather than as a patho-genetic influence.

CONCLUSIONS AND IMPLICATIONS

American social work has been increasingly conscious of the cultural factors in individualized and group services. Dealing with generations of immigrants and their children, group workers have also experienced in their relationships with clients the significance of the differences in cultural background. It is our position that group work practice with Asian clients is a part of social work practice with a sociocultural orientation. We also believe that a special emphasis in practice is needed where cultural factors are involved besides the general "group work principles."

In discussing the process of entering group treatment, it is important to examine the process from the perspective of the Asian client's role expectations of the worker. The worker is often perceived as an authority figure and is respected as such. Awareness of the potentially complex multi-generational transferences to the group leader can lead to creative, flexible, and sensitive group interventions, depending on the leader's goals and the capabilities of the Asian group members. Taking a more directive approach in the group process is generally the expected course of action for the group worker. However, such an approach can be significantly modified as the Asian group members evolve and as their expectations of the group leader change. It is possible then to transit slowly to a less directive, less authoritarian stance over time. The role of family members must also be understood and the proper respect for their influences on group members is essential for a positive group treatment.

As indicated earlier, most Asians have a different attitude toward the open sharing of feelings and problems from that of Americans. For instance, the process of face saving has its early origin in child rearing practices, which use group pressures of the family and peers. These methods induce shame to punish non-conforming behavior.

Cultural norms hold the family responsible for the individual's behavior. The shame for the individual's behavior is experienced by the family and extended even to the family's ancestors.

The burden of the shame and stigma of mental illness, traditionally has fallen on the family and the individual. The psychotic individual's bizarre and non-conforming behavior brings much shame and guilt onto the family. Many families, to avoid "losing face," tend to deny the existence of mental illness, or attempt to cover up the unacceptable behavior with somatic or medical problems. This shame and stigma have been the primary reasons for avoiding mental health services and a critical impediment to successful psychotherapy. In our experiences, a special effort should be made for a great deal of education and delicate restructuring before group members feel comfortable enough to express their feelings openly. The worker should also be sensitive to nonverbal cues in the group such as changes in facial expressions or tone inflections. The initiation of self-disclosure and open exploration of feelings in a group setting with Asian clients would be facilitated by the active attempts of the group leader to promote the psychological transformation of the group from a "non-family" or "public" identification into a "family" identification. Once Asian group member see themselves as being within a "family" setting, there is significant release of tension. Concerns about loss of face, though still present, do not carry the associated fears of abandonment and loss of support, and the non-public aspects of the self should slowly appear among Asian group members.

It should be realized that because "Asian-American" represents such a variation in Asian sub-cultural groups, it is difficult for a social worker to know how best to help an Asian client. However, the social worker's role in working with Asian groups will be that of a culture broker and enabler, helping and guiding group members to recognize their own sociocultural values and to resolve their conflicts or dysfunction. According to Shon and Ja (1982), an Asian worker is generally preferable in working with Asian clients because of the complexities of Asian cultures and family systems. We further support their view that a culturally sensitive non-Asian worker is preferable to an insensitive Asian. A key element in the group process is the ability of the non-Asian workers, for instance, to explore their feelings and stereotypes about Asian-Americans in general and Asian clients in particular and the willingness to develop their own potential to become a source of cultural enrichment.

While there may be cultural differences in the manner Asians and non-Asians present or express their problems in group therapy, it has to be recognized that Asians in groups also behave in some basic patterns that vary little from non-Asians.

For example, groups, whether Asian or non-Asian, tend to depend on the leader to scapegoat or displace aggression on the weakest members of the group, and group members tend to be influenced by their family histories.

Resistances to deal with the work of the group are also common to all groups. Although the Western values emphasize the value of revealing one's problems and the Eastern values emphasize the concern with saving face, all members of a group defend themselves in varying degrees from experiencing public humiliation and shame. All groups use periods of silence and intellectual defenses, for example, to avoid revealing sensitive material or strong affects.

Group leaders of all groups need to understand the effect their authority roles as change agents play in the group process. When the group leader is perceived by the group as another "member of the family," it could facilitate group acceptance but could also subtly neutralize the leader's authority. If the leader does not interpret this process after the initial "acceptance phase," the collusion can nullify the leader's ability to complete the treatment task.

As with all groups, the group leader must deal with the multiple levels of complexity involving the overt and covert processes, the conscious and the unconscious, the individual dynamics, the interpersonal, and the group phenomena.

It is the authors' hope that this brief analysis of some of the sociocultural factors in group interventions with Asian clients will contribute toward a better understanding of the problems and stimulate a wider interest in their application.

REFERENCES

Chang, C.C. Experiences with group psychotherapy in Taiwan. *International Journal of Group Psychotherapy*, 1972, *22* (2), 210-227.

Chew, A.K. Treatment implications of cultural attitude toward dependency/independency. In. W. Ishikawa & N. Archer (eds.) *Service delivery in Pan Asian communities.* San Diego: Pacific Asian Coalition, 1975.

Dio, T. *The anatomy of dependence.* New York: Harper & Row, 1973.

Fujii, A. Elderly Asian Americans and use of public services. *Social Casework*, 1976, *57* (3), 202-207.

Garvin, C.D. *Contemporary group work.* Englewood Cliffs, N.J.: Prentice-Hall, Inc. 1981.

Ho, M.K. Social work with Asian Americans. *Social Casework*, 1976, *57* (3), 195-201.

Hong, L.K., & Tsukashima, R.T. (Eds.). Asian/Pacific Americans. *California Sociologist,* 1980, *3* (2), 76-230.

Kaneshige, E. Cultural factors in group counseling and interaction. *The Personnel and Guidance Journal,* 1973, *51* (6), 407-412.

Kim, B.L. Casework with Japanese and Korean wives of Americans. *Social Casework,* 1972, *53 (5),* 273-279.

Kim, B.L. Asian American: No model minorities. *Social Work*, 1973, *18* (3), 44-53.

Kim, B. L. *The Asian Americans: Changing patterns, changing needs.* Montclair, N.J.: Association of Korean Christian Scholars in North America, Inc., 1978.

Kitano, H.L. (Ed.). *Asians in America.* New York: Council on Social Work Education, 1971.

Kleinman, A., & Lin, T.Y. (Eds.). *Normal and abnormal behavior in Chinese culture.* Boston: D. Reidel Publishing Co., 1980.

Kuramoto, F. What do Asians want? An examination of issues in social work education. *Journal of Education for Social Work*, 1971, *7* (3), 7-17.

Lum, D. et al. The psychosocial needs of the Chinese elderly. *Social Casework*, 1980, *61* (2), 100-106.

Matsushima, N.M., & Tashima, N. *Mental health treatment modalities of Pacific/Asian American practitioners.* San Francisco: Pacific Asian Mental Health Research Project, 1982.

Montero, D., & Dieppa, I. Resettling Vietnamese refugees: The service agency's role. *Social Work*, 1982, *27* (1), 60-67.

Morales, A. Social work and third-world people. *Social Work*, 1981, *26* (1), 45-51.

Murase, K. (Ed.). *Asian American task force report: Problems and issues in social work education.* New York: Council on Social Work Education, 1973.

Northen, H. *Social work with groups.* New York: Columbia University Press, 1969.

Ozawa, M. Social welfare: The minority share. *Social Work*, 1972, *17* (3), 32-43.

Ryan, A.S. Training Chinese-American social workers. *Social Casework*, 1981, *62* (2), 95-105.

Salcido, R.M., Nakano, G., & Jue, S. The use of formal and informal health and welfare services of the Asian-American elderly: An exploratory study. *California Sociologist*, 1980, *3* (2), 213-219.

Shon, S.P., & Ja, D.Y. Asian families. In M. McGoldrick et al. (Eds.), *Ethnicity and family therapy.* New York: The Guilford Press, 1982.

Stern, L.M. Response to Vietnamese refugees: Surveys of public opinion. *Social Work*, 1981, *26* (4), 306-311.

Sue, S., & McKinney, H. Asian-American clients in the community mental health system. *American Journal of Orthopsychiatry*, 1975, *45* (1), 111-118.

Sue, S., & Sue, D.W. Chinese-American personality and mental health. In Sue & Wagner (Eds.), *Asian American psychological perspectives.* California: Science and Behavior Books, 1973.

Toupin, E.A. Counseling Asians: Psychotherapy in the context of racism and Asian American history. *American Journal of Orthopsychiatry*, 1980, *50* (1), 76-86.

Yamamoto, J. Therapy for Asian Americans. *Journal of the National Medical Association*, 1978, *70* (4), 267-270.

Social Group Work
with Asian/Pacific-Americans

Man Keung Ho

ABSTRACT. This paper discusses the Asian/Pacific clients and the group practice modality. Specific suggestions are offered to help group workers better understand Asian/Pacific-American clients, capitalize on their unique strengths, and minimize their limitations. Part I of this paper addresses practical group work considerations for the Pre-Group Phase; Part II addresses practical group work considerations for the Group Interaction phase.

This paper discusses the Asian/Pacific-American client and the group practice modality. Specific suggestions are offered to help group workers better understand Asian/Pacific-American clients, capitalize on their unique strengths, and minimize their limitations. The ultimate objective is to improve service and provide greater benefits to this ethnic minority. The mental health and social service needs of Asian/Pacific-Americans have been documented by various authors (Kim, 1973; Abbott and Abbott, 1973; Endo, 1974). There is also clear evidence that this group under-utilizes mental health services and social services (Sue and McKinney, 1975). This under-utilization can often be attributed to the service provider's insensitivity to the client's help-seeking orientation (Tseng and McDermott, 1975).

While a few articles outlining culture-sensitive approaches in working with Asian/Pacific-Americans have appeared (Ishisaka and Takagi, 1982; Shon and Ja, 1982; Ho, 1976), there is no literature that specifically addresses and provides practical guidelines in the use of group as a practice modality in providing services to this

Man Keung Ho, PhD, is Professor of Social Work, University of Oklahoma.

49

ethnic group. This paper presents practical guidelines in using group as a practice modality in providing services to Asian/Pacific Americans. These guidelines should be augmented with a sensitive awareness of Asian/Pacific-American historical and cultural background and theoretical material that other publications can provide (e.g., Sue and Morishima, 1982; Wong, 1982; Green, 1982).

Because of the traditional help-seeking behavior on the part of the Asian/Pacific-American who prefers problems (interpersonal and psychological) to be resolved within the famiy (Lin et al., 1978; Lin and Lin, 1978), the use of an "artificial" or "formed" group as a practice modality is debatable. However, the purpose of this paper is not to debate or make general statements about the appropriateness or irrelevance of the use of group with Asian/Pacific-Americans; rather it explores ways group mobility can best be utilized to maximize the benefits and services of Asian/Pacific-American clients. Cultural issues are reviewed and practical guidelines in using the group modality are specified. For clarity the paper is divided into two sections: Part I addresses practical group work considerations for the Pre-Group Phase; Part II addresses practical group work considerations for the Group Interaction Phase.

PART I: PRACTICAL CONSIDERATIONS
FOR THE PRE-GROUP PHASE

Selection of Candidates for Groups

The effectiveness and power of a group depends to a large degree on who participates. According to the philosophical democratic assumptions of Social Group Work set forth by Coyle (1959), the "traditionalist" Asian/Pacific-Americans who are early immigrants and the recent arrivals may find group interaction intimidating, confusing and, therefore, non-productive. The American-born of any generation are more likely to display acculturated behaviors reflecting their socialization in the United States and, therefore, may find group interaction more responsive to their needs. Moreover, American-born individuals, who understand majority systems and have less reason to distrust professional services may find group interaction enriching.

Hence, a client's acculturation and adaptation in the United States usually determines the degree to which the client can benefit from group interaction. There are four criteria to determine a client's degree of acculturation (Lee, 1982): (1) Years in the United States: as a whole, the longer the client lives in the States, the more he or she is acculturated; (2) Age at time of immigration: an 8-year-old is more easily assimilated than an 80-year-old; (3) Country of origin, political, economic, and educational background: a Chinese graduate student from Hong Kong (British Colony) is more easily assimilated than a young adult from Mainland China; (4) Professional background: an English-speaking Japanese doctor is more easily assimilated than a Japanese cook.

While American-born individuals may be prospective candidates for a group requiring more intensive interaction, the non-native Asian/Pacific-American can take advantage of a concrete task group or an educational group focusing more on information giving and less on the exchange of personal opinions and feelings. Kim (1978) points out that the non-native client's initial requests for service tend to be predominantly requests for information and referral, advocacy, and such other services as English-language instruction, legal aid, and child care.

Client's Conceptions of Group Purposes

Since purpose usually denotes the specific reason(s) for which the group is formed and expresses the type of goals that the group will try to help its members attain, the group purpose or objective needs to be carefully phrased. The traditional social work treatment of remedial groups implicating individual failure or disfunctioning may alienate prospective Asian/Pacific-American group members or cause them to terminate prematurely. Asian/Pacific-Americans find it difficult to admit they have emotional or psychological difficulties, because such problems arouse considerable shame and a sense of having failed one's family. They will respond more favorably should they perceive the group purpose as an obligatory means to meet their concrete basic needs such as employment, food, and shelter. Their acceptance of such group purposes is consistent with their traditional social explanation to disorienting events (Green, 1982). This type of explanation allows the individual to see himself or herself as a victim of some unfortunate but uncontrollable events, a result of nonpersonal determinants.

Group purpose(s) emphasizing the rehabilitation of physical or organic illness also is acceptable to Asian/Pacific-American clients.

As a matter of fact, organic explanations for personal dysfunction are most common in Asian/Pacific culture (Kleinman and Lin, 1981). The client's preference for "impersonal" physical illness excuses moral failure and familial irresponsibility.

Client's Expected Behavior in Group

A group worker should be cognizant of how an Asian/Pacific American may interact in a group. For a group member to benefit from group therapy, he or she usually believes in the "therapeutic" process characterized by the client's acceptance of the problem, the need, and motivation for change (Garvin, 1981). Individual group members also believe that long-range goal setting and the process of "working through" are essential to correct past defective experiences. Verbal, intimate, emotional, self-disclosing, and behavioral feedback are seen as central to the change process (Yalom, 1975).

In contrast, Asian/Pacific-American group members may find it difficult to accept the fact that they have problems and may feel they haven't tried hard enough to overcome them. If the problem continues to cause pain, clients develop a fatalistic attitude and bear the problem in stoic fashion (Ho, 1976). Asian/Pacific group members are deterred from directly confronting other group members because they have been taught that it is rude to put people on the spot. Free participation and the exchange of opinions in a group also contradict Asian values of humility and modesty. "Don't be a show-off or engage in any behavior that smacks of being a braggart," is a common Asian admonition, and it is directly responsible for assigning Asian/Pacific-Americans silent-member roles in a group.

"Reactivation of early childhood experience," a popular concept in Western group therapy (Yalom, 1975) cannot be expected of Asian/Pacific-American group members. Asian/Pacific Americans perceive themselves minimally important as compared to the importance of their families. The individual exists and is important only in relation to his/her family. Thus, the public exposure of family conflicts in the process of resolving individual conflicts and eventually achieving self-fulfillment is an unacceptable display of selfishness and exaggerated self-importance (Kaneshige, 1973). During the group process, the worker should keep in mind these basic differences of Asian/Pacific Americans and guard against unreasonable expectations of these clients.

Client's Expectations of Worker's Role in Group

Most Asian/Pacific-Americans fail to understand the role of a group worker and may confuse him/her with a physician. They always regard the worker as the knowledgeable expert who will guide them in the proper course of action. Hence, the group worker is seen as an authority figure and is respected as such. The client expects that the authority figure will be more directive than passive. Being directive does not mean that the worker should tell the clients how to live their lives. It does involve directing the process of the group session. A group worker needs to convey an air of confidence. When asked, he/she should not hesitate to disclose personal educational background and work experience. Asian/Pacific-American clients need to be assured that their worker is more powerful than their illness or problems and will "cure" them with competence and know-how.

Some Asian/Pacific-American clients may ask the worker many personal questions about family background, marital status, number of children, and so on. The worker will need to feel comfortable about answering personal questions in order to gain a client's trust and to establish rapport. Once trust and rapport with the worker is established, clients may form a dependency on the worker. It would be a mistake to assume that such overtures or apparent dependency patterns necessarily indicate tranference of other difficulties. Given the interpersonal complexity of Asian/Pacific cultures, forming relationships that mirror those found in family groups or in friendship networks may be helpful to the client as a means of guiding the interpersonal process with the worker (Green, 1982).

Due to the strong emphasis on obligation in Asian/Pacific culture, clients may consider keeping appointments or following directives as doing something for the worker in return for the worker's concern. The worker should neither condemn nor confront such client behavior but capitalize on it to help the clients resolve their problems (Ho, 1982).

Homogeneous vs. Heterogeneous Group Composition

Heterogeneous grouping involving various sub-groupings should be avoided in view of Asian/Pacific-Americans' cultural characteristics that discourage admission of failure and personal problems, free expression and confrontation. Having to communicate in

English adds an additional stress. Whenever possible Asian/Pacific-Americans of a particular nationality and geographical location should be grouped together. Chinese from Hong Kong should be grouped separately from Chinese from Taiwan or American-born Chinese. The clear need for such categorical groupings is commonality in sub-culture and language efficiency essential for group progress and the achievement of group goals. Should all members meet the language requirement, in that they all speak fluently the same dialect or the English language, heterogeneous grouping with various sub-groups from the same country or nationality is acceptable. Workers should be very cautious about composing a group across various nationalities of Asian/Pacific-American origins. Despite their common Asian/Pacific historical and cultural backgrounds, strong feelings of prejudice and nonacceptance among much of the Asian/Pacific population still exist. Fewer communication and cultural barriers will be experienced in heterogeneous groups if all members are American-born respective of any generation.

Asian/Pacific-American interpersonal interaction revolves around a vertical and hierarchical role structure which is determined by age, sex, generation, and birth order of family members. Cross sex and generation groupings are therefore discouraged. Generally, the more traditional (culture) the member is the less desirable for him or her to be included in a heterogeneous group. An acculturated member should experience less difficulty in a cross-sex or cross-generation group interaction characterized by an egalitarian relationship and mode of interaction.

Culturally-Relevant Group Structure

The vertical and hierarchical role structure which forms an Asian/Pacific American's early relationship patterns with others also influences how such clients interact in a group work situation. The group's basic structure should clearly define the worker in a leadership role. Should a group worker fail to assume a leadership role, especially at the beginning stage of a group, a high drop-out rate among Asian/Pacific group members is to be expected. Cultural traits such as strong will, discipline, deference, and loyalty toward an authority figure (worker) generally have a positive effect on Asian/Pacific-American clients and enhance their ability to function as strong group members. These clients may refuse to be a part of an organization and a group that lacks structure. Asian/Pacific-Americans will tend to perceive such a group as irrelevant, unpractical, lacking leadership, direction, strength, and hope.

Asian/Pacific-American clients' expectation of a vertical group structure in which the worker assumes a leadership role should not be misconstrued as their unresponsiveness to the mutual aid system concept. The key issue is "how," on the part of the worker, to facilitate the members in helping one another to achieve their individual and collective aspirations. The worker needs to assume a more direct and active role especially at the beginning stage of a group. As the group progresses, members feel more secure and comfortable with each other, realizing each has strengths to aid others in solving problems rather than each depending solely on the worker. Only then can a more egalitarian relationship be facilitated to maximize fully the usefulness of the group as a problem-solving modality.

Preparing Members for the Group

The idea that members, who are prepared for the group experience are more likely to benefit from it, is receiving increased support (Northen, 1969; Yalom, 1975). Preparation is particularly essential for the Asian/Pacific-American client who has no prior experience in a problem-solving group. To prepare an Asian/Pacific client for the group, the worker needs to perform the following functions:

1. Describe to the client in concrete terms how a group can be used for problem solving. If it is feasible, the worker can play a portion of a video tape highlighting the value and application of the group process.
2. Point out to the client the importance of honest interpersonal exploration, including open expression and disclosure of inner feelings for problem solving. It is vital that the worker solicit feedback from the client at this time and explain carefully to the client that discomfort and uneasy feelings are experienced by all members especially at the beginning of a group.
3. Share with the client that fear and discouragement are common feelings experienced by group members, and that problem-solving is a gradual process that takes time and endurance.

4. Share with the client that the worker is mindful of the anxiety and discomfort the client may experience and that the client can always choose not to be an active participant, such as being on the "hot seat" or the focal point of group discussion. Further, the client can always count on the worker's support during moments of uncertainty and stress.
5. Assure the client that everything that transpires in the group will be confidential.
6. Explain to the client that the worker's role is different from that of a physician and describe some of the specific activities the worker will perform in the group.

Properly preparing Asian/Pacific-American clients prior to their participating in a group is an essential step and one a worker should always consider when dealing with this specific ethnic group. Careful preparation will reduce the drop-out rate of Asian/Pacific-American clients and help them maximize the group process. When all the pre-group tasks have been completed, the worker can proceed to the group interaction phase.

PART II: PRACTICAL CONSIDERATIONS FOR GROUP INTERACTION PHASE

The Role of the Worker

A group worker must recognize that he/she is being a model for all group members, but especially so for Asian/Pacific-Americans who value authority. The worker's tone of voice and manner of interaction with each group member are unconsciously, and sometimes consciously, noted and may do much to encourage or stifle verbal expressiveness. Additionally, a worker needs to pay attention to interpersonal grace with warm expressions of acceptance, both verbally and nonverbally. The worker can do this, for instance, by asking about the client's health, offering a cup of tea, suggesting the client remove his/her coat, or indicating a more comfortable chair. Such expressions serve to convey genuine concern and can add greatly to beginning and maintaining a positive relationship (Green, 1982).

While it is important for the worker to assume an authoritarian role in terms of providing directions for interaction, especially at the beginning of a group, he/she also needs to convey an air of support and consideration to the group. For instance, the worker can comment on the cultural value differences and the apparent internal struggle that the Asian/Pacific-American group member faces. The worker can assist the verbally "non-expressive" and "non-assertive" Asian/Pacific-American group member who is struggling for self expression by minimizing interruptions from other group members. During the beginning phase of the group, the worker should avoid constant direct eye contact with Asian/Pacific-American clients who may interpret it as a challenge or confrontation.

Asian/Pacific cultures place high value on what others think of them. The worker should make a special effort to help Asian/Pacific-American clients avoid disgracing themselves in public. For instance, prior to asking an individual in front of the group if he/she has successfully completed a contract (obligation), the worker needs to be sure that a negative answer will not make the client feel publicly disgraced. In addition, whatever the worker can do to enhance the individual's acceptance by the group will be reciprocated by Asian/Pacific-American clients who view externally derived evaluations as a part of one's system of self (Norbeck and DeVos, 1972).

Structured Short-Term Concrete Goals

The ability of Asian/Pacific-American clients to utilize group service for problem solving depends largely on their country of origin, length of stay, socio-economic status and facility in English. Recent arrivals and more long-term residents who lack fluency in the English language usually will not seek or be receptive to group services. Those who are American-born or of long residence in the United States are more likely to seek help for personal matters or difficulties, and they are generally receptive to the use of a group as a problem-solving modality.

In spite of their acceptance of group service, most Asian/Pacific-American clients find loosely targeted and abstract long-term goals incomprehensible, unreachable, and impractical. Instead, they prefer structured and goal-directed work with clear and concrete objectives (Murase and Johnson, 1974). A group worker should not rule out the possibility, however, that some Asian/Pacific clients may respond well to highly personalized therapy focused on emotional areas. Recipients of this therapeutic work should be carefully selected and it should not be attempted without a strong worker/client trusting relationship.

Culturally Relevant and Strength-Focused Skills and Techniques

The pragmatic nature of Asian/Pacific cultures coupled with the client's unfamiliarity with Western "talk therapy" and the English language make insight-oriented therapies and techniques (Psychoanalytic-oriented therapy, existentialism, and Gestalt therapy) irrelevant and non-productive to Asian/Pacific clients. In contrast, structured, strong-willed, goal-directed short-term practice theories or therapies with clear and concrete objectives—such as Crisis Intervention, Task-Centered, Behavioral Therapy, and Rational Emotive therapy—are more relevant and responsive to the Asian/Pacific-American client's need for problem solving. Short-term cognitive behavioral-oriented practice theories tend to focus less on the client's past relationship with parents and make neither the client nor the parents the frequent target of group concern or the subject for group sharing. Behavioral-focused therapy challenges the client's motivation for filial piety (change for the better and for the parents). It also challenges the client's will power to modify that specific segment of behavior that causes shame and alienation.

The Asian/Pacific-American client's strong sense of obligation can be capitalized on in group work. The worker's warm acceptance of clients can make them feel they should be mutually accepting of the worker. The worker can use the clients' feelings of obligation to return favors to challenge the clients to follow instructions or directives and to help with the group. The worker can ask Asian/Pacific-American clients to assist other members who need help. Such concrete services can include providing transportation for other group members, making physical arrangements for group meetings, and providing tea or coffee for the group. By providing the group worker and the group such concrete services, Asian/Pacific-American clients feel needed. Through validation and positive evaluation from others, their self-esteem improves and interpersonal problems become manageable. Asian/Pacific Americans also value loyalties, including the loyalty that develops between the client and the worker and the client with other clients. Such loyalty encourages regular group attendance and fosters group cohesiveness. Thus, the strength and positive group traits demonstrated by Asian/Pacific-American clients can serve as a stabilizing force for group cohesiveness in ethnic, heterogeneous groups.

Asian/Pacific Americans are sensitive toward others who care about them and know them, including group members. Confrontative techniques, generally recognized as essential rools for unmasking psychological defense and resistance, are often counter-productive with Asian/Pacific-American clients. They highly value what others think of them and usually take criticism as a personal attack, an unacceptable insult, and an interpersonal rejection. If Asian/ Pacific clients need to be confronted about their impasse or persistent resistance responsible for their dysfunctional behavior, the worker should refrain from a *direct* confrontation with the clients. Moreover, the worker should stop others in the group from directly attacking the client. Instead, the worker can use an "indirect" means to help clients encounter their problems. For instance, if a client continues to defy his employer in a passive-aggressive manner, the worker should help the client recognize the difficulty by commenting, "I wonder what others (outside the group) will say about 'our' behavior if they learn what 'we' did." Without directly assigning the Asian/Pacific-American client a specific directive for improving relationships with others, the worker may endorse such behavior and get the group to endorse it also. For example, the worker can remark, "I might politely let my employer know that somehow I see the same thing differently than he does." The Asian/ Pacific-American client usually is perceptive and will test new directives (behavior). By reporting the success of a new behavior to the group, the client gets an opportunity to be re-affirmed by others in the group.

The use of role-playing by volunteering members, video-playback of role-playing, group discussions, and other graphic and visual aids can facilitate the group process with Asian/Pacific-American clients.

Evaluation and Termination

Considering the Asian/Pacific client's deference to an authority figure and unreadiness for verbal participation in the group, a spontaneous and honest feedback of worker intervention is unrealistic. An innovative method of assessment which takes into consideration the client's cultural background is best for Asian/Pacific-American clients. Such evaluative methods should be systematic but anonymous, focusing on the worker's employment of relevant means or procedures in helping the clients resolve individual and group goal(s) or problems (Ho, 1980).

The process of termination should also consider the Asian/

Pacific-American client's concept of time and space in relationship. The client may regard the group worker as a family member and may want to maintain contact with the group worker even after the successful achievement of treatment goals. For many Asian/Pacific-Americans, a good relationship is a permanent one that should be treasured.

Individual Conference as a Supplement

In view of the Asian/Pacific-American client's general unfamiliarity with group work, high degree of tolerance, and restrictive verbal participation in the group, periodic individual conferences should be scheduled regularly with each group member. The main purpose of individual conferences is to ascertain if the client is benefiting from the group process. During the conference, which usually lasts between 10 to 15 minutes, the worker can offer support and specific suggestions to the client regarding expected behavior in future group sessions. It is important that the worker refrain from exploring with the client an issue or problem(s) that best be dealt with in the group. The worker's attention and time spent with each client in individual conferences will reduce the drop-out rate and enrich client interaction and results in the group.

CONCLUSIONS

Asian/Pacific-American clients' unfamiliarity with social group work in no way implies that they are deprived of early group experience, or that they cannot benefit by group as a service modality. The interdependent and collective nature of their culture has not fully prepared them to interact and make the most of group experiences. The challenge is for group workers to familiarize themselves with cultural and historical Asian/Pacific backgrounds. For effective group interaction, workers should adapt relevant techniques and skills in working with these clients. Generally, group process resembling the Asian/Pacific-American family interaction and friendship network appeals most to Asian/Pacific-American clients and can provide the most benefit.

This presentation represents only the author's observations based on a review of current literature and direct work with this ethnic group. Empirical studies are needed that delineate and specify indications and contra-indications of group work practice with Asian/Pacific-Americans.

REFERENCES

Abbott, K. A., and Abbott, E. L. Juvenile delinquency in San Francisco's Chinese-American community: 1961-1966. In S. Sue and N. N. Wagner, eds., *Asian-Americans: Psychological perspective*. Palo Alto, Calif.: Science and Behavior Book, 1973.

Coyle, G. Some basic assumptions about social group work. In M. Murphy ed., *The social group work method in social work education, 2,* 88-105, 1959.

Endo, R. Japanese Americans: The model minority in perspective. In R. Gomez, C. Cottingham, Jr., R. Endo, and K. Jackson, eds., *The social reality of ethnic America.* Lexington, Mass.: D.C. Heath, 1974.

Garvin, C. *Contemporary group work.* Englewood, N.J.: Prentice Hall, 1981.

Green, J. *Cultural awareness in the human services.* Englewood, N.J.: Prentice-Hall, 1982.

Ho, M. K. Social work with Asian-Americans. *Social Casework, 57,* 195-201, 1976.

Ho, M. K. A model to evaluate group work practice with ethnic minorities. Paper presented at the 1980 *Social Work with Group Symposium*, Arlington, Texas, 1980.

Ho, M. K. Building on the strengths of minority groups. *Practice Digest, 5,* 6-7, 1982.

Ishisaka, H., and Takagi, C. Social work with Asian and Pacific Americans. In J. Green ed., *Cultural Awareness in the Human Services.* Englewood, N.J.: Prentice-Hall, 1982.

Kaneshige, E. Cultural factors in group counseling and interaction. *Personnel and Guidance Journal, 51,* 407-412, 1973.

Kim, B. D. Asian-Americans—No Model Minority. *Social Work, 18,* 44-53, 1973.

Kleinman, A., and Lin, T.Y., eds.. *Normal and deviant behavior in chinese culture.* Hingham, Mass.: Reidel, 1981.

Lee, E. A social systems approach to assessment and treatment for Chinese American families. In M. McGoldrick, et al., eds., *Ethnicity and family therapy.* New York: Guilford Press, 1982.

Lin, T., and Lin, M.L. Service delivery issues in Asian North American communities. *American Journal of Psychiatry, 135,* 454-56, 1978.

Lin, T.K., Donetz, T.G., and Goresky, W. Ethnicity and patterns of help seeking. *Culture, Medicine and Psychiatry,* 213-13, 1978.

Murase, T., and Johnson, F. Naikan, Morita and Western psychotherapy. *Archives of General Psychiatry, 31,* 1974, 121-28.

Norbeck, E., and Devos, G. A. Culture and personality: The Japanese. In Hsu, F.L. ed. *Psychological Anthology in the Behavioral Science.* Cambridge, Mass.: Schenkman, 1972, 21-70.

Northern, H., *Social work with groups.* New York: Columbia University Press, 1969.

Son, S., and Davis, J. Asian families. In M. McGoldrick, et al., eds., *Ethnicity and family therapy.* New York: Guilford Press, 1982.

Sue, S., and McKinney, H. Asian-Americans in the community mental health care system. *American Journal of Orthopsychiatry, 45,* 111-18, 1975.

Sue, S., and Morishima, J. *The mental health of Asian-Americans.* San Francisco: Jossey-Bass, 1982.

Tseng, W.S., and McDermott, J.T. Psychotherapy: Historical roots, universal elements and cultural variations. *American Journal of Psychiatry, 132,* 378-84, 1975.

Wong, H.Z. Mental health services to Asian- and Pacific-Americans. In L. Snowden, ed., *Services to the underserved.* Los Angeles: Sage Reviews of Community Mental Health, 1982.

Yalom, I. *The theory and practice of group psychotherapy* (2nd ed.). New York: Basic Books, 1975.

Call for Papers

Contributions are invited for a special issue of *Social Work with Groups.* The special issue is to appear in the Fall of 1986 and will be devoted entirely to research in group work. Special guest editor will be Ronald A. Feldman of Washington University, St. Louis. Associate guest editors are Larry E. Davis, (Washington University, St. Louis), Maeda Galinsky (University of North Carolina, Chapel Hill), Sheldon D. Rose (University of Wisconsin, Madison), Martin Sundel (University of Texas, Arlington) and James K. Whittaker (University of Washington, Seattle).

Consideration will be given to research reports, evaluations of group work programs, synthesis of research concerning pertinent practice topics, discussions of research advances or methodological issues, operationalization of dependent and independent variables in group work practice or research, the study of group developmental processes, and analyses of measurement issues or techniques. Original papers on any and all aspects of group work research are welcome.

All manuscripts should conform to the requirements of manuscripts for *Social Work with Groups.* Papers can be submitted to the Special Editor for this issue at The George Warren Brown School of Social Work, Washington University, St. Louis, Missouri 63130. While the deadline for submission is December 1, 1985, manuscripts will be welcome in advance of that date.

The Utility of Group Work Practice for Hispanic Americans

Frank X. Acosta
Joe Yamamoto

ABSTRACT. This article examines the utility of group work practice for Hispanic Americans who represent the second largest ethnic minority group in the United States. Special focus is given to the utility of group work practice with Hispanics who are primarily unacculturated and predominantly monolingual Spanish-speaking. A number of reports on group work practice with Hispanics are considered and several important clinical issues and problems in group work practice with Hispanics are discussed. The role of both training and experience for therapists and the consideration of cultural factors in conducting group work are discussed and seen as crucial for effectiveness. The use of behavioral and experiential approaches and the use of short-term and long-term approaches are seen as successful and valuable treatment alternatives when applied in appropriate contexts in group work practice with Hispanics.

INTRODUCTION

The Hispanic population in the United States is at least 12 million, with the Mexican-American group showing the largest subpopulation (U.S. Bureau of the Census, 1980). In Los Angeles

Frank X. Acosta is Associate Professor of Clinical Psychiatry, Department of Psychiatry and the Behavioral Sciences, University of Southern California, School of Medicine Los Angeles, California. Joe Yamamoto is Professor of Psychiatry, Neuropsychiatric Institute, University of California, Los Angeles.

Preparation of this manuscript was assisted by Grant MH27899-05 from the National Institute of Mental Health Center for Prevention Research, Division of Prevention and Special Mental Health Programs.

Address correspondence to Frank X. Acosta, PhD, Department of Psychiatry and the Behavioral Sciences, University of Southern California School of Medicine, 1934 Hospital Place, Los Angeles, California 90033.

County alone, the population of the Hispanic community is 2.0 million, or 28.7 percent of the County's entire population (Los Angeles County, 1978).

A number of studies have clearly demonstrated that in spite of their long history in this country, Hispanic Americans face a number of serious social, economic, and political needs and pressures (LeVine and Padila, 1980; Acosta, Yamamoto and Evans, 1982). Substantial evidence has affirmed that the majority of Hispanic Americans are a disadvantaged group and find themselves greatly behind the larger society in total amount of education, occupational status, income, housing, political representation, and professional identification. In addition to these life stressors, Hispanic Americans have further experienced difficulties in encountering language barriers with their strong reliance on Spanish and in dealing with the process of acculturation to the United States (Acosta, 1979). It has been demonstrated, for example, that Hispanics have shown the longest nurturance and maintenance of a language other than English, compared to other ethnic minority groups in this country.

While information is still lacking, it is believed that the levels of psychological distress and the incidence of psychological disorders due to the heavy life stressors encountered by Hispanic Americans are probably high among the Hispanic Americans and particularly among the unacculturated Hispanics (Acosta, 1977; Yamamoto and Acosta, 1982). Unfortunately, the stigma of mental illness, and the clouding by this stigma of those mental health services which may be available, continues to be a deterrent and a problem in effectively providing mental health services to the Hispanic community. For those Hispanics who have made the brave decision to seek help in our adult psychiatric outpatient clinic based on a referral by a family member, a physician, a social agency or on their own, we do see a wide range of severe psychological problems. The largest percentages of psychiatric disorders that patients are presenting include major affective disorders, adjustment disorders, and schizophrenic disorders.

The focus of this article will be on the utility of group work practice approaches for Hispanics who are primarily unacculturated and predominantly Spanish-speaking. This group of Hispanics probably represents the greatest challenge to clinicians and represents individuals with the most severe needs.

THE USE OF GROUP WORK PRACTICE WITH HISPANICS

Over the past two decades a small number of reports have discussed the use of group work practice with Hispanic patients. One of the earliest reports on group practice with Hispanics by Maldonado-Sierra and Trent (1960) described the use of specific therapist roles for three co-therapists who enacted Puerto Rican characteristics of an older sibling, a father, and a mother in the group treatment of chronic, regressed male schizophrenic Puerto Rican patients. Both successes and failures among individual patients were reported by the authors.

During the 1970s a number of unique approaches with primarily Puerto Rican- and Mexican-American patients are described. These will be briefly illustrated. Normand, Iglesias, and Payne (1974) found encouraging results in implementing time-limited therapy as the initial treatment for Spanish-speaking patients. This approach marked a clear demarcation from the more usual practice of conducting at least brief individual therapy prior to initiating group psychotherapy.

Philipus (1971) reported an innovative effort to make clinical services more available to the Mexican-American community. The group practice approaches which Philipus reported included both Anglo and Mexican-American patients of varying degrees of English fluency. When English rather than Spanish was the language used more in the group, Mexican-Americans were found to show much higher drop-out rates.

The treatment of a Mexican-American woman by a specialized intervention for distressed adult Mexican-American women was reported by Heiman, Burruel, and Chavez (1975). In their approach both environmental interventions and traditional psychotherapy were successfully applied. The use of county transportation to bring Spanish-speaking patients to a group was reported as central to their efforts by Hynes and Werbin (1977). These authors reported that this unique outreach effort was essential to maintain the group since patients could not otherwise have attended. The group was found to be successful in helping patients deal with their loneliness and with their severe somatic distresses.

The use of a behavioral group approach in the treatment of Spanish-speaking Mexican-American men and women was reported as successful by Herrera and Sanchez (1976). In addition, Boulette

(1976) found in a study which compared assertiveness training with non-directive psychotherapy that Mexican-American women showed greater gains in self-esteem and in assertiveness through the assertiveness training group. Both of these studies point to the potential usefulness for behavioral approaches with Hispanic patients.

A small number of reports in the 1980s have to date supplied additional understanding to the usefulness of group work practice with Hispanics. LeVine and Padilla (1980) have recently reported favorable results in a number of studies reviewed on group conseling with Hispanic children, adolescents, and young adults. The use of weekend encounters and of participation by Hispanics in multi-ethnic groups were noted to be positive experiences for the Hispanic participants.

The experimental study of a control, a cognitive therapy, and a behavior therapy group approach was recently reported by Comas-Diaz (1981). In this study it was found that low-income Puerto Rican women who participated in either cognitive group therapy or in behavior group therapy showed significant reductions in depression compared to the control patients who received no immediate treatment. No significant differences were found between the behavior and cognitive group approaches. This study, together with the study by Boulette (1976), represents one of the few empirically designed group work studies with Hispanics.

The use of group work practice as reported in the literature does strongly indicate that more successes than failures are encountered in implementing group services for Hispanic patients.

CLINICAL ISSUES IN GROUP WORK PRACTICE

Appropriateness of Patient for Group Treatment

In facilities which do not have significant numbers of bilingual or Spanish-speaking staff clinicians, it is very easy for non-Spanish-speaking therapists to refer patients with very different diagnostic difficulties to Spanish-speaking groups. In an effort to be helpful it is tempting for a Spanish-speaking clinician to accept the majority of referrals if the clinician has an ongoing group program. Such a process was our own experience until very recently.

We had felt a clinical mandate to accept Spanish-speaking patients to existing Spanish-speaking groups with minimal screening. This has proven to be very difficult for both therapists and patients involved in group treatment. It is particularly difficult, for example, to conduct group treatment with patients who are suffering primarily from neurotic or adjustment disorders if a patient also participates who is suffering from either active paranoic ideation or psychotic symptomatology. This often causes distress for the majority of the patients who may be either in good remission from previous psychotic experiences or who may be anxious or depressed individuals.

It has further proven to be extremely difficult to conduct group work if a patient participating is predominantly suffering from a narcissistic and demanding personality in addition to a particular life crisis or other neurotic symptoms. Such patients have been found over the years to be highly disruptive to the group process. For example, these patients may dominate a group session, then return the following session with a new problem never having resolved or taken action on the previous problem. It is certainly challenging to try to teach a narcissistic patient group courtesy and protocol, but such a patient often proves to erode the group spirit of other patients and also proves exhausting to group therapists.

Problems in Group Composition and Patients' Reactions

It is important for group therapists working with Hispanic and Spanish-speaking patients to consider the variety of issues involved in the composition of a group. For example, it has proven to be difficult to conduct a group if there are significant class differences among the patients. It has often been problematic for poorly educated patients to understand and to communicate easily with more highly educated and upper-class patients. It has also been found that the more highly educated upper-class patient is less accepting of the poor and less educated patient.

As already discussed, the factors of diagnostic homogeneity or heterogeneity are important issues for therapists to weigh. During the past year the staff clinicians in our clinic have experimented with the concept of establishing more homogeneous groups based on patient diagnosis. Such groups as the neurotic disorders group, the affective disorders group, and the thought disorders group have been conducted in the past year and are meeting with good success.

The authors have found that there has been no problem in enrolling patients with different Hispanic backgrounds into the same group. On occasion there have been strong clashes between patients, but these have been related more to the patients' personalities than to their ethnic origin. Thus, groups have been effectively conducted with Hispanic patients from Mexican-American, Central American, Cuban-American, and Puerto Rican-American backgrounds.

The sex of a patient is a further important issue to consider in composing a Spanish-speaking group or a Hispanic group. We have found that more women than men accept and participate in group practice: The ratio has often been 3 to 1 in favor of women. Men have also been much more reluctant to speak openly in group settings.

Just as Hispanic patients are typically not familiar with mental health treatment, they are even less familiar with group treatment. It is important to recognize this lack of familiarity and to be sensitive to the patient's understanding of group process. This is particularly important in the initial sessions of treatment. We have encouraged patients to explain their experiences to new members and have found this to be an important model. If patients have been reluctant to explain their experiences with group treatment to new patients, therapists have initiated this explanation and have continued to encourage patients to do so. The importance and utility of preparing patients for mental health services and for continually educating patients has been strongly recommended by Acosta, Yamamoto, and Evans (1982).

Problems may be encountered by group therapists: When some patients feel a lack of individual attention from the therapist, they may become resentful. This is particularly so if a patient does not realize immediate progress for his/her own particular problems. Often it is not possible for problems to be resolved quickly within the group format since time is obviously shared by all of the members. It is thus important for therapists to be sensitive to this potentially negative reaction by patients. The therapist should further be sensitive to the patients potential fear of self-revelation or disclosure within a public forum. In brief, the therapist should pay particular attention to the needs and unique fears and concerns of the new patient entering group therapy.

THERAPIST'S TRAINING AND EXPERIENCE

It is important to note that therapists cannot simply assume that their skills learned in individual practice may be easily transposed to group work practice. The unique processes which occur in the group setting and the stressful, at times, requirements for effective group leadership definitely require specialized training in conducting group work. These issues have been cogently examined by McCarley, Yamamoto, Steinberg, and Anker (1983). These authors have argued that a group therapist should be thoroughly trained by participating in didactic seminars which focus on group dynamics and group process, group observations by observing through either a one-way mirror or through being seated in the actual group, co-therapy training, practical experience, supervision, and personal group experience.

It is often most helpful, either in training or in actual practice, to conduct group work with a co-therapist. In either case, whether working with a peer or with a supervisor, it is critical for a therapist to explore his or her personal reactions in a non-defensive and open fashion to experiences occurring within the group and to the therapist's reactions to the group as a whole or to individual patients within the group. In addition, reactions occurring within oneself or with one's co-therapist should be openly discussed. It is easy for clinicians who are very busy to conduct a group as co-therapists and not discuss ther personal reactions to their group experience which they may have. It is further crucial for co-therapists to be clear about their own roles within the group and about the direction of treatment for the group and for each patient in the group.

In the authors' experience in training group therapists, it has been discovered that trainees often express the uniqueness of their experience in working with Hispanic and Spanish-speaking patients and the personal reward which they experience in working with Hispanics in group process. It has further been gratifying to see trainees who initially may be very reluctant about their own language fluency in Spanish, quickly overcome their reluctance and improve their fluency. Patients have been consistently accepting of therapists with Spanish language limitations and have consistently helped with language clarification if a therapist is limited in Spanish.

As part of training for group work practice with Hispanics, the emphasis is on the cross-cultural and cross-ethnic dimensions of treatment within the Hispanic population. For both ethnic minority and non-ethnic minority therapists, a great challenge is to continue to improve one's sensitivity and knowledge about the cultural background and current milieu of patients (Acosta et al., 1982).

Special Cultural Considerations

In the authors' experience it has been found that it is important to recognize that such cultural factors as religion, family networks, and acculturation have potentially powerful impacts on a Hispanic patient (Acosta, 1982; Yamamoto and Acosta, 1982). It is important for therapists to assess the role, for example, of religion in the life of a particular Hispanic patient. It may be that religion is playing either a large or a small role in a patient's quest for relief from psychological suffering. The role of the patient's family and friends in either providing support or creating distress for a patient should further be evaluated. It is often that the assumed strength of a Hispanic patient's family network is not present for the patient who is seeking psychiatric help. For those patients whose families are intact, whether they are in conflict or not, attempts to involve family members with the patient outside of group work for explanation and support to the patient's treatment course are also made.

GROUP WORK PRACTICE APPROACHES

Short-Term Groups

The authors have found that the use of short-term contracting with patients in a newly forming group can be highly effective. Unfortunately, it is much harder to initiate and conduct a short-term group with all patients beginning at the same time. Often the clinical demands of mental health facilities call for groups to be ongoing to some degree and it is often difficult to identify an adequate core of new patients quickly enough to begin a new group for short-term treatment only. A fair amount of time and energy is often required in establishing an adequate core number of patients to begin a short-term group. It is difficult then for therapists to continually repeat the process of recruiting new patients to start a new short-term group.

As a compromise to the difficulty of continually initiating a new group, the authors have modified the usefulness of short-term group process to contract for short-term treatment with many of the new patients entering ongoing groups. They have found that when Hispanic patients begin treatment it is often more appealing for them to think in terms of briefer periods of treatment time. To this end the authors have been successful in securing a *compromiso* or commitment from a patient for a short-term treatment plan in group. They have found that the drop-out rates from group work practice have been reduced dramatically.

Furthermore, the authors have found that ongoing patients of groups adapt well to the process of multiple changes in group composition. Here, new patients enter into treatment or former patients terminate from treatment. This process is somewhat akin to that described by Normand et al. (1974) as earlier discussed. These experiences in themselves often stimulate a great deal of previously unresolved experiences for some patients and a new forum for trying new behaviors in both meeting new individuals and in the often painful experience of terminating relationships.

Long-Term Groups

For some patients it is essential to offer them long-range treatment based on their individual psychological problems. The authors have found, for example, that patients with long-standing personality or neurotic difficulties will not be amenable to short-term change. Often Hispanic patients will be offered treatment on a short-term basis to resolve more immediate and pressing difficulties or crises. If appropriate and necessary, long-term group treatment for more chronic difficulties will then be offered. It is often more immediately known for patients suffering from psychotic disorders that they will need longer-term treatment to maintain their progress. For these patients it is explained at the onset of their treatment in group work that their treatment will be of a longer range nature for their own well-being. This explanation is often accepted well by patients who understand the scope of their problem.

Group Process

Patients are encouraged in group work to assume greater responsibility for their own treatment. This phenomenon has often proved provocative for new patients entering group work and the authors have found it necessary to both encourage and explain the importance of patient participation in the power and direction of their own group treatment. It is nonetheless difficult for Hispanic patients to accept this concept of group sharing and responsibility for treatment, and patients often expect the therapist to assume more of an authoritative or parental role.

The authors have found it productive to combine both behavioral and experiential approaches in group treatment. In addition, they have encouraged patients participating in group to be highly involved in helping patients to solve environmental pressures and problems in daily living. Patients have been found to be very compliant in completing specific homework assignments to be conducted outside of group. The reporting of behaviors attempted or discussions held with significant others outside of group have been meaningful to patients in recognizing their own participation in treatment.

CONCLUSION

In this article the authors have considered how group work practice may be a viable and important approach to help meet some of the mental health needs for Hispanic Americans. Based on the authors' clinical experience and on a review of the efforts by others, it strongly appears that the often neglected Hispanic and Spanish-speaking-only patient may benefit a great deal from group work practice. We have recommended, however, that before a patient is invited to a particular group, the therapist consider such patient characteristics as sex, socioeconomic status, and level of acculturation. Also to be considered are the patient's diagnoses, personality characteristics, and treatment needs to assure the best possible fit between the patient and the group.

It has proven to be particularly effective to provide early educational explanations to Hispanic patients about the process of group work practice. In addition, where possible, it has further proven to be an advantage to provide short-term group treatment and to encourage patients to make a *compromiso* or a commitment to their own progress.

In conclusion, it has been the authors' experience that group work practice for Hispanic Americans is a valuable treatment approach and is also an ongoing forum for new knowledge and new challenges.

REFERENCES

Acosta, F. X. Ethnic variables in psychotherapy: The Mexican American. In J. L. Martinez (ed.), *Chicano Psychology*. New York: Academic Press, 1977, 215-231.
Acosta, F. X. Barriers between mental health services and Mexican-Americans: An examination of a paradox. *American Journal of Community Psychology*, 1979, 7, 503-520.

Acosta, F. X. Group psychotherapy with Spanish-speaking patients. In R. M. Becerra, M. Karno, & J. I. Esocobar (eds.), *Mental Health and Hispanic Americans*, 1982, pp. 183-197.

Acosta, F. X., Yamamoto, J., & Evans, L. A. *Effective psychotherapy for low-income and minority patients*. New York: Plenum Publishing Corp., 1982.

Boulette, R. T. Assertive training with low-income Mexican-American women. In M. R. Miranda (ed.), *Psychotherapy with the Spanish-speaking: Issues in research and service delivery*. Monograph 3. Los Angeles: Spanish Speaking Mental Health Research Center, University of California, 1976, 67-72.

Comas-Díaz, L. Effects of cognitive and behavioral group treatment on the depressive symptomatology of Puerto Rican women. *Journal of Consulting and Clinical Psychology*, 1981, *49*, 627-632.

Heiman, E. M., Burruel, G., & Chavez, N. Factors determining effective psychiatric outpatient treatment for Mexican-Americans. *Hospital and Community Psychiatry*, 1975, *26*, 515-517.

Herrera, A. E., & Sanchez, V. C. Behaviorally oriented group therapy: A successful application in the treatment of low-income Spanish-speaking clients. In M. R. Miranda (ed.), *Psychotherapy with the Spanish-speaking: Issues in research and service delivery*. Monograph 3. Los Angeles: Spanish Speaking Mental Health Research Center, University of California, 1976, 73-84.

Hynes, K., & Werbin, J. Group psychotherapy for Spanish-speaking women. *Psychiatric Annals*, 1977, *7*, 622-627.

LeVine, E. S., & Padilla, A. M. *Crossing cultures in therapy: Pluralistic counseling for the Hispanic*. Monterey, CA: Brooks/Cole, 1980.

Los Angeles County. *Population report Los Angeles County*. (Evaluation, research & statistics report No. F-640). Los Angeles: County of Los Angeles Department of Health Services, 1978.

Maldonado-Sierra, E. D., & Trent, R. D. The sibling relationship in group psychotherapy with Puerto Rican schizophrenics. *American Journal of Psychiatry*, 1960, *117*, 239-244.

McCarley, T., Yamamoto, J., Steinberg, A., & Anker, M. V. Teaching group psychotherapy. In M. Grotjahn, F. M. Kline, C. T. H. Friedmann (eds.), *Handbook of Group Therapy*. New York: Van Nostrand Reinhold Co., 1983, pp. 195-210.

Normand, W. C., Inglesias, J., & Payne S. Brief group therapy to facilitate utilization of mental health services by Spanish-speaking patients. *American Journal of Orthopsychiatry*, 1974, *44*, 37-42.

Philipus, M. J. Successful and unsuccessful approaches to mental health services for an urban Hispano American population. *American Journal of Public Health*, 1971, *61*, 820-830.

U.S. Bureau of the Census. *Statistical abstract of the United States: 1980 (101st ed.)*. Washington, D.C.: U.S. Government Printing Office, 1980.

Yamamoto, J., & Acosta, F. X. Treatment of Asian Americans and Hispanic Americans: Similarities and differences. *Journal of the American Academy of Psychoanalysis*, 1982, *10*, 585-607.

Content Themes
in Group Treatment
with Puerto Rican Women

Lillian Comas-Díaz

ABSTRACT. This paper discusses an empirical observation of the thematic content in a cognitive-oriented group treatment. Clients were low socioeconomic Puerto Rican women who were assessed as depressed. Preliminary findings indicate that the discussed themes included interpersonal relations, children, spouse, mental symptoms, family of origin, and culture shock. Such themes bear a relationship to Puerto Rican cultural values such as *personalismo* and *marianismo*. The author concludes that group practice is applicable and effective when treatment is linguistically and culturally syntonic with the needs of Puerto Rican clients.

Myths surrounding the lower socioeconomic class clients imply that they are not amenable to traditional clinical treatment (Jones, 1974). These clients have been described as distrustful of the clinician, limited in self-observation, and lacking the capacity for verbal communication (Weissman and Klerman, 1973). In a statistical sense, most minority clients receive supportive or mechanical treatment more often than traditional clinical ones (Cole and Pilsuk, 1976). Moreover, the minority individual in treatment has been subjected to bias and stereotyping. As a consequence, the efficacy of clinical treatment for this population has been questioned. Smith, Burlew, Mosley and Whitney (1978), state that minority clients in treatment are easily stereotyped because they are treated by clinicians representative of Anglo middle-class values who do not understand them. This situation leads to the need for research in clinical practice which is aware of and attempts to minimize effects of socioeconomic, class, ethnic, race, and gender bias.

Puerto Ricans are a low-income, ethnic minority group in the

Lillian Comas-Díaz, PhD is in the Department of Psychiatry at Yale University, New Haven, CT.

75

United States. They have to struggle with the effects of migration, poverty, plus linguistic and cultural barriers. Due to their minority group membership they are at risk of psychological distress and may therefore benefit from clinical treatment. Indeed, Acosta (1979) states that the difficulties which can ensue due to socioeconomic and acculturation pressures could create a high need for mental health services among Hispanics.

Additionally, these individuals have to cope with disruptions in cultural routines and attacks on cultural values; thus, the ethnic identity is threatened. A correlation between conflicts in ethnic identity and resultant psychological stress has been suggested. Individuals who are in the midst of cultural change can experience problems with ethnic identity, while those who have strong dual identities may experience less conflict around identity (Baynard, 1978). Acculturation may further erode the psychological well-being of the Puerto Rican client. Fernandez-Pol, (1978) in her empirical research, found that Puerto Ricans of lower socioeconomic classes who adhered to Latin American family values had less psychopathology than Puerto Ricans who were more acculturated. Subsequently, it could be inferred that Puerto Ricans who have strong dual identities, or those who adhere to traditional cultural values, seem to have more effective coping mechanisms.

Another stressor for Puerto Ricans is culture shock. Culture shock has been defined as the set of emotional reactions to: the loss of reinforcements from one's own culture, new cultural stimuli which have little or no meaning, and the misunderstanding of new and diverse experiences (Adler, 1980). It may also be accompanied by feelings of helplessness, irritability, and rejection. Similarly, Ruiz (1975) states that a loss of self-esteem and a sense of powerlessness characterize members of minority groups who are trying to cope with the culture shock that follows migration. Garza-Guerrero (1974) asserts that culture shock is accompanied by a process of mourning brought about by the individual's loss of family, friends, language, and culturally determined values and attitudes. He further adds that culture shock causes a threat to the individual's identity and that the mourning process might lead to depression.

Depression is identified as a major problem among mainland Puerto Ricans (Normand, Iglesias and Payn, 1974). Specifically, the Puerto Rican woman seems to be more prone to depressive reactions than the Puerto Rican man (Abad and Boyce 1979). She is socialized into a non-assertive, dependent, and traditionally feminine position (Silén, 1972). According to Klerman and Weissman (1980) traditional female roles may contribute to depression. In regard to the effectiveness of clinical practice for low socioeconomic and ethnic minority clients, group treatment has proven to be a relevant modality. Strupp and Bloxom (1975) have used it successfully while developing a role induction film to prepare lower class clients for group modality. Likewise, Ruiz (1975) states that group work practice helps ethnic clients to gain insight into their personality conflicts. Moreover, Maldonado-Sierra and Trent (1960) found that when group treatment was made culturally relevant to Puerto Rican clients, it proved to be beneficial. They focused attention upon the sibling relationship in the treatment. In the same manner, Hynes and Werbin (1977) used group modality with Hispanic women, incorporating into the group the challenge of cultural variables such as the men's *macho* role, the meaning of fatalism, and the use of magic as a sole resource, among others. They found that group practice was successful with Hispanic women who were feeling oppressed, helpless and depressed.

There is a dearth of empirical exploration in clinical work with Puerto Ricans. There is virtually no quantitative description of the content themes in clinical treatment: what clients actually discuss in treatment. This paper presents preliminary clinical impressions of the treatment content with Puerto Rican women. It explores the content themes in a short-term group treatment with depressed Puerto Rican women who had migrated to the United States mainland.

METHODOLOGICAL APPROACH

Clients were eight low socioeconomic class Puerto Rican women who were referred to a community mental health center for treatment of depression by local social service agencies. They were Puerto Rican-born women, middle age (mean age of 36, with a range of 27 to 44), unmarried, and living with children. Clients had an average of six years of education. All women were raised as Catholics. They were unemployed and received some form of governmental aid. They were monolingual in Spanish and had an average of five years of residence in the United States mainland, interrupted by migration and reverse migration to and from the island. The clinician had a session with perspective participants at a social service agency in order to discuss their pre-treatment expectations.

In addition, the purpose and method, as well as the duration of the treatment, were explained to them.

The assessment of depression was made by self-report, using the Spanish version of the Beck Depression Inventory (Comas-Díaz and Santiago, 1978a), clinical ratings using the Spanish version of the Hamilton Rating Scale (Comas-Díaz and Santiago, 1978b), and by a depression rating scale (Comas-Díaz, 1981). Participants in this group treatment carried diagnoses ranging from adjustment reactions with depressive features to depressive neuroses. Women thought to be psychotic, demented, addicted to drugs, or severely suicidal were not accepted for this treatment, but were referred to another form of treatment.

The group treatment followed Beck's (1967) cognitive theory. Torres-Matrullo (1982) asserts that cognitive techniques are an effective and applicable approach to the treatment of depression among Hispanic clients, specifically Hispanic women. She states that this approach is effective in dealing with unrealistic, culturally-based expectations regarding male and female sex-role behaviors. Cognitive treatment is a directive, active, time-limited structured approach (Beck, Rusk, Shaw, and Emery, 1978). The clinician followed a protocol developed by Shaw (1975) of a cognitively oriented group treatment for depression. Treatment included exploration, examination, confrontation, and modification of depressive cognitions. Treatment, conducted in Spanish, lasted for five 1-1/2-hour sessions and was audiotaped. The clinician was a female Puerto Rican (author).

The method of scoring used for the content themes was devised by Weissman, Paykel, and Prysoff (1972). The content themes included physical symptoms, mental symptoms, current treatment, practical problems, family of origin, spouse (or lover), sex, children, interpersonal relations, and early experiences. For the purpose of this empirical exploration, another category was added: culture shock, which was operationally defined as any verbalization around migration, feelings about the new country, conflict in cultural values, and sociocultural adjustment problems.

PRELIMINARY FINDINGS

All themes were rated by time present during the session on the following scale: 0 (none)—less than 3 minutes; 1 (brief)—3 to 5 minutes; 2 (moderate)—6 to 15 minutes; 3 (sustained)—over 15 minutes cumulative time (Weissman and Klerman, 1973). The clinician rated the five audiotaped sessions. Another Hispanic clinician rated two sessions selected at random in order to assess reliability of scoring. There was a 93 percent rate of agreement between the two raters. All content themes were scored for the five sessions. The total scores for each content theme during the five sessions were added. The percentage of group sessions where the various content themes were discussed either briefly or not at all were rated (0 or 1), moderately or sustained (rated 2 or 3); these ratings were calculated for the five sessions. The frequency of themes discussed by clients is shown in Table 1.

All the women participated actively in discussing themes. While the majority of the themes were discussed, there was a variation in the amount of time spent on each theme. Clients discussed the following themes in a moderate or sustained manner: interpersonal

Table I

Frequency of content themes discussed during
the five sessions of group treatment

Time present in sessions*

Content Themes	Not at all or briefly (rated 0 or 1); % of sessions	Moderately or sustained (rated 2 or 3); % of sessions
Interpersonal Relations	20%	80%
Children	20%	80%
Spouse/Lover	40%	60%
Mental Symptoms	40%	60%
Family of Origin	40%	60%
Culture Shock	60%	40%
Current Treatment	60%	40%
Physical Symptoms	80%	20%
Early Experiences	80%	20%
Practical Problems	100%	0%
Sex	0%	0%

* 0 (None)   Discussion lasted less than 3 minutes.
  1 (Brief)   Discussion lasted 3 to 5 minutes.
  2 (Moderate) Discussion lasted 6 to 15 minutes.
  3 (Sustained)Discussion lasted over 15 minutes.

relations, children, spouse (lover), mental symptoms, family of origin, culture shock, and current treatment. Physical symptoms, early experiences, and practical problems were discussed only briefly while sex was not discussed at all.

DISCUSSION

Traditional group treatment can be an effective and beneficial means of treatment for low socioeconomic ethnic minority women. The outcome study of the effectiveness of this cognitive group treatment is discussed elsewhere (Comas-Díaz, 1981). Women participated actively in their treatment and were involved in exploring content themes that are usually thought of when considering involvement in treatment: interpersonal relations, children, spouse (lover), family of origin, mental symptoms, and current treatment.

The cognitive treatment orientation may have encouraged and/or limited the expression of certain themes. Within the cognitive framework, depression is perceived in terms of a set of three cognitive patterns that force the person to view himself/herself, his/her world, and his/her future in an idiosyncratic way (Beck, 1967). The depressed person sees himself/herself as inadequate and deficient, experiences his/her reality in a negative way, and finally anticipates his/her situation will continue indefinitely. According to this model, depressive cognitions include a low self-regard, ideas of deprivation, self-criticism, overwhelming problems and duties, self-blame, self-commands and injunctions, plus escapist and suicidal wishes (Beck, 1967). Cognitive treatment delineated the systematic modification of maladaptive patterns of thinking. Examination, evaluation, and modification of negative cognitions are also included (Beck, Rusk, and Shaw, 1978). During treatment the client needs to explore the origin of negative cognitions and resort to earlier experiences. Therefore, the cognitive treatment may have encouraged the expression of themes related to the negative cognition such as symptoms (mental and physical), relationships with significant others (interpersonal relationships, children, spouse/lover), and early experiences. On the other hand, this approach may have limited the expression of themes not related to the treatment style.

The preliminary findings suggest that group modality is a relevant treatment for Puerto Rican women clients. Group work practice is consistent with several Puerto Rican cultural characteristics

(Maldonado-Sierra and Trent, 1960). Moreover, a group treatment with Hispanic women seems to have additional therapeutic effects (Hynes and Worbin, 1977), hence, a Puerto Rican women's group has unique advantages. For instance, Wolf (1952) states that lower socioeconomic class Puerto Rican women in an all-female group format discuss topics such as feelings about womanhood and anger toward significant others (husbands, children, parents, etc.) which, culturally, are not allowed to be expressed directly. This practice, closely related to Puerto Rican cultural values, may have contributed to the early development of a collective sense of identity in the group.

Puerto Rican cultural values can also help to explain the prevalence of some content themes over others during the group treatment. The Puerto Rican culture ascribes importance to personal relationships. In fact, the cultural concept of *personalismo* emphasizes the personal quality of any transaction or interaction. Therefore, *personalismo* may explain the high incidence of discussion of interpersonal relations. Moreover, the high frequency of discussion around children and spouse (lover) can be attributed to the cultural value of *marianismo*. This concept, based on the cult of the Virgin Mary, states that women are to be self-sacrificing toward their children and endure the suffering inflicted by men (Stevens, 1973). For example, statements such as, "being a mother is the highest task in life," "our children always come first," "a woman who is a mother is closer to God," were enunciated by some women and received unanimous support from the group members.

The sustained discussion of culture shock is of significant relevance. Alder (1975) proposes a developmental model of culture shock following different stages. This model suggests that specific psychological, cultural, and social dynamics appear during culture shock. The model delineates a progression through five stages: (1) contact, where a person is insulated by his or her culture; (2) disintegration, where awareness of being different results in depression and withdrawal; (3) reintegration, where the second culture is rejected through anger and rebellion, thus asserting one's self and increasing self-esteem; (4) autonomy, where the person is able to culturally negotiate different situations, hence are assured of surviving new experiences; and (5) independence, where social, psychological, and cultural differences are accepted and enjoyed (1975). Clients in the present treatment expressed feelings characteristic of the disintegration stage, where growing awareness of being different leads to loss of self-esteem, confusion, withdrawal, and depression. Although the women had an average stay of five years on the mainland United States, such feelings seem to result, at least partially, from constant migration between Puerto Rico and the mainland. Clients discussed issues around migration, cultural conflicts, and adjustment difficulties. Although migration has been identified as a crisis in transition among the general population (Fried, 1964), for lower socioeconomic class minority individuals the crisis is accentuated in moving to an environment where the majority group is in control of major institution and prejudice and stereotyping will occur. This finding suggests that the clients might be dealing with a depressive reaction experienced by Puerto Ricans who are coping with changes in cultural and social values (Trautman, 1961).

In the present exploration the discussion of physical symptoms was not prevalent. These findings are not consistent with the high incidence of somatic complaints reported by Puerto Rican clients (Abad and Boyce, 1979). Moreover, Hynes and Werbin (1977) assert that among Hispanic women reporting somatic complaints is a way of obtaining support from significant others. It can be speculated that group treatment can address and modify this behavior. Sex was the only topic that was not discussed. There are several possible explanations for this finding. Within the Puerto Rican culture women discussing sex in public is taboo. Cultural norms discourage the image of a woman as a sexual being. Another variable that might have inhibited the discussion of this topic is the short length of the treatment. Five sessions were not sufficient for the development of *confianza* (trust that requires a long time to develop) in order to discuss cultural taboos like sex.

This empirical observation reveals that although practical problems were discussed during treatment sessions, they were not discussed in a sustained manner. These findings are not consistent with Weissman and Klerman's study in that they found that depressed women in treatment discussed practical problems in a sustained manner. Several variables can be responsible for this difference. In Weissman and Klerman's (1973) investigation the clinicians followed an individual treatment model "aimed at identifying maladaptive patterns and attaining better levels of adaptive response." Moreover, treatment lasted eight months. The present exploration followed a cognitive group format and treatment lasted five sessions. These variables might be accountable for the difference in results.

The present exploration shows that depressed Puerto Rican women can participate actively in group treatment. This suggests that group work practice may be a treatment modality relevant for this population. It also suggests that the clinician's lack of bias against this type of population in treatment is of great importance. The clinician was from the same culture, race, gender, and was familiar with the low socioeconomic life style. This common ground seemed to facilitate the women's participation in therapy.

The sustained discussion of topics such as children, spouse (lover), and interpersonal relations suggests that these issues are relevant for Puerto Rican women. The high frequency of discussion of these themes may also suggest that cultural values such as *marianismo* and *personalismo* may need to be addressed in working with this population. Moreover, the high frequency of discussion of issues relating to culture shock among clients indicates that treatment with depressed Puerto Rican women should include coping skills to deal with the culture shock. Indeed, in a recent review of group treatment with Spanish-speaking clients, Acosta (1982) indicates that a recurring theme in clinical practice involves the stress of adapting to a different society. He asserts that group practice can be very effective with Hispanics who are feeling alienated, lonely, and depressed. Similarly, this empirical observation suggests that group treatment is applicable and effective with Hispanic clients if and when the treatment is linguistically and culturally syntonic with the unique needs of this population.

REFERENCES

Abad, V. & Boyce, E. Issues in psychiatric evaluations of Puerto Ricans: A socio-cultural perspective. *Journal of Operational Psychiatry,* 1979, 10, 28-39.

Acosta, F.X. Barriers between mental health services and Mexican-American: An examination of a paradox. *American Journal of Community Psychology,* 1979, 7, 502-520.

Acosta, F.X. Group psychotherapy with Spanish-speaking patients. In R. Becerra, M. Karno, & J.I. Escobar (eds.), *Mental Health* and *Hispanic Americans: Clinical Perspectives.* New York: Grune & Stratton, Inc., 1982, 183-197.

Adler, P. The transitional experience: An alternative view of culture shock. *The Journal of Humanistic Psychology.* 1975, 15, 4, 13-23.

Bayard, M.P. Ethnic identity and stress: The significance of sociocultural context. In J.M. Casas and S.E. Keefe (eds.), *Family and mental health in the Mexican-American community.* Los Angeles: Spanish-speaking Mental Health Research Center, University of California, 1978.

Beck, A.T. *Depression: clinical, experimental, and theoretical aspects.* New York: Harper and Row, 1967.

Beck, A.T., Rusk, A.J., Shaw, B.F. & Emery, G. *Cognitive therapy of depression: A treatment manual.* Unpublished manuscript (available from A.T. Beck, Department of Psychiatry, University of Pennsylvania, Philadelphia, Pa.), 1978.

Cole, J. & Pilisuk, M. Differences in the provision of mental health services by race. *American Journal of Orthopsychiatry,* 1976, 46, 3, 510-525.

Comas-Díaz, L. & Santiago, N.I. Spanish version of the Beck Depression Inventory. Unpublished manuscript, (available from L. Comas-Díaz, Department of Psychiatry, Yale University, 690 Howard Ave. New Haven, CT 06519) 1978 A.

Comas-Díaz, L & Santiago, N.I. Spanish version of the Hamilton Rating Scale. Unpublished manuscript (available from L. Comas-Díaz, Department of Psychiatry, Yale University, 690 Howard Ave., New Haven, CT 06519) 1978 B.

Comas-Díaz, L. Effects of cognitive and behavioral group treatment on the depressive symptomatology of Puerto Rican women. *Journal of Consulting and Clinical Psychology,* 1981, 49, 5, 627-632.

Fernandez-Pol, B. Culture and psychopathology: A study of Puerto Ricans. *American Journal of Psychiatry,* 1980, 137, 6, 724-726.

Fried, M. Social problems and psychopathology. In Group for advancement of psychiatry (eds.), *Urban Americans and Mental Health Planning.* New York: GAP, 1964.

Garza-Guerrero, A.C. Culture Shock: Its mourning and vicissitudes of identity. *Journal of the American Psychoanalytic Association,* 1974, 22, 408-429.

Hynes, K. & Werbin, J. Group psychotherapy for Spanish-speaking women. *Psychiatric Annals,* 1977, 7, 12, 52-63.

Jones, E. Social class and psychotherapy: A critical review of research. *Psychiatry,* 1974, 37, 307-320.

Klerman, G. & Weissman, M. Depressions among women: Their nature and causes. In M. Guttentag, S. Salusin, & E. Belle (eds.) *The mental health of women.* New York: Academic Press, 1980.

Maldonado-Sierra, E. & Trent, R. The sibling relationship in group psychotherapy. *American Journal of Psychiatry,* 1960, 117, 3, 239-244.

Normand, W., Iglesias, J., & Ryan, S. Brief group therapy to facilitate utilization of mental health services by Spanish speaking patients. *American Journal of Orthopsychiatry,* 1974, 44, 1, 37-49.

Ruiz, P. Symposium: Group therapy with minority group patients. *The International Journal of Group Psychotherapy.* 1975, 25, 4, 389-390.

Shaw, B.A. *A systematic investigation of two psychological treatments of depression.* Doctoral dissertation, University of Western Ontario, Ontario, Canada, 1975.

Silén, F. *Hacia una visión positiva del puertorriqueño.* Rio Piedras, Puerto Rico: Editorial Edil, 1972.

Smith, W.D., Burlew, A., Mosley, M., & Whitney, W. *Minority issues in mental health.* Reading, Mass.: Addison-Wesley Publishing Company, 1978.

Stevens, E. Machismo and marianismo. *Transaction/Society,* 1973, 10, 6, 57-63.

Strupp, H. & Bloxom, A. Preparing lower-class patients for group psychotherapy: Development and evaluation of a role induction film. In M. Rosenbaum & M. Berger (eds.) *Group psychotherapy and group function.* New York: Basic Books, 1975, 658-671.

Torres-Matrullo, C. Cognitive therapy of depressive disorders in the Puerto Rican female. In R. Becerra, M. Karno, & J.I. Escobar (eds.) *Mental Health and Hispanic Americans: Clinical Perspectives.* New York: Grune and Stratton, Inc., 1982, 101-113.

Trautman, E. Suicidal attempts of Puerto Rican immigrants. *Psychiatric Quarterly,* 1961, 35, 4, 544-554.

Weissman, M.M., & Klerman, G.L. Psychotherapy with depressed women: An empirical study of content themes and reflection. The British Journal of Psychiatry, 1973, 123, 572, 55-61.

Weissman, M., Paykel, E.S., & Prusoff, B. Checklist qualification of a psychological therapy: Pilot studies of utility. *Journal of Nervous Mental Disease,* 1972, 154, 125-136.

Wolf, K. Growing up and its price in three Puerto Rican subcultures. *Psychiatry,* 1952, 15, 4, 401-433.

Hispanics and Group Work:
A Review of the Literature

Melvin Delgado
Denise Humm-Delgado

ABSTRACT. This article reviews the literature on group work with Hispanics and highlights key practice issues and considerations. A total of 28 publications are analyzed with reference to such elements as group member and leader characteristics and possible facilitating factors.

INTRODUCTION

The use of group work to meet the needs of Hispanics in the United States has been extensively explored by human service providers in a variety of geographical and practice settings. This method of intervention is economical and can be practiced in virtually any setting, address a multitude of needs and, in some instances, be the treatment of choice. Further, it is culturally acceptable if undertaken within a culturally sensitive environment.

Although the professional literature is rich with references to the use of group intervention with Hispanics, a systematic review of the literature has not been undertaken; thus, this article reviews 28 manuscripts published since 1970 and highlights key practice issues and considerations.*

The article is organized in three sections: group characteristics, practice issues, and conclusions. First, a section on group characteristics is based upon the 17 publications that describe actual groups. Second, practice issues in the literature regarding conduct-

---

Melvin Delgado, PhD, is Associate Professor, Boston University School of Social Work, Boston, MA. Denise Humm-Delgado, PhD, is Assistant Professor, Simmons College, School of Social Work, Boston, MA.

*Please see Reference Note for source of articles.

ing groups with Hispanics are delineated, based upon all 28 publications (both empirical and theoretical). Third, conclusions are drawn from the total literature.

GROUP CHARACTERISTICS

The 17 articles that describe groups provide an overview of some of the group work that has been successfully utilized with an Hispanic clientele in the past several years. These articles are examined in terms of five aspects: (1) location, (2) type and scheduling of group, (3) language usage, (4) participant characteristics, and (5) leader characteristics.

Location

A review of the geographical locations of the authors shows that New York and California are the sites of most of the groups described. Nine articles describe group efforts in New York City (Cooper and Hernandez-Cento, 1977; Franklin and Kaufman, 1982; Kraidman, 1980; Leon, 1981; Menikoff, 1979; Normand, Iglesias, and Payn, 1974; Richmond et al., 1977; Rodriguez, 1971 [this article describes a group just outside of New York City]; Tylim, 1982). Six articles originate in California: in Los Angeles (Acosta, 1982; Herrera and Sanchez, 1976; Koegler and Williamson, 1973), San Mateo (Hynes and Werbin, 1977; Werbin and Hynes, 1975), and San Francisco (Maduro, 1976). Two articles also originate in Massachusetts: in Worcester (Delgado and Siff, 1980) and Framingham (Hardy-Fanta and Montana, 1982).

Mental health settings are the most usually cited for Hispanic groups. Outpatient mental health groups are cited in ten of the 17 articles (Acosta, 1982; Franklin and Kaufman, 1982; Herrera and Sanchez, 1976; Hynes and Werbin, 1977; Koegler and Williamson, 1973; Kraidman, 1980; Leon, 1981; Menikoff, 1979; Normand, Iglesias, and Payn, 1974; Werbin and Hynes, 1975). Inpatient (Rodriguez, 1971) and day hospital and treatment (Richmond et al., 1977; Tylim, 1982) are other mental health settings utilized. A university (Maduro, 1970) and schools (Delgado and Siff, 1980; Hardy-Fanta and Montana, 1982) are also sponsors of groups. Lastly, one article concerns a group (prenatal) in a medical department of a hospital (Cooper and Hernandez-Cento, 1977).

Type and Scheduling of Group

Three-quarters (13 of 17) of the groups provided group therapy— four of a long-term nature (1-5 years) and with a stable membership (Franklin and Kaufman, 1982; Kraidman, 1980; Menikoff, 1979; Werbin and Hynes, 1975), two of a short-term nature (Hardy-Fanta and Montana, 1982; Normand, Iglesias, and Payn, 1977), two open-ended but with a changing membership (Koegler and Williamson, 1973; Tylim, 1982), and five of a length not specified in the publication. Three other groups are described as support groups (Cooper and Hernandez-Cento, 1977; Delgado and Siff, 1980; Leon, 1981) and one as a socialization group (Rodriguez, 1971).

Few of the articles indicate the length of time scheduled for group sessions. However, when indicated, 1-½ hours is the most frequently mentioned (Franklin and Kaufman, 1982; Hynes and Werbin, 1977; Koegler and Williamson, 1973), followed by one hour (Cooper and Hernandez-Cento, 1977; Tylim, 1982), and 1-1/4 hours (Herrera and Sanchez, 1976) and three-quarters of an hour (Delgado and Siff, 1980).

Language Usage

When noted, Spanish was the language of choice in Hispanic groups (Acosta, 1982; Cooper and Hernandez-Cento, 1974; Franklin and Kaufman, 1982; Herrera and Sanchez, 1976; Hynes and Werbin, 1977; Kraidman, 1980; Koegler and Williamson, 1973; Leon, 1981; Menikoff, 1979; Normand, Iglesias, and Payn, 1974; Rodriguez, 1971; Tylim, 1982; Werbin and Hynes, 1975). However, an article that deals with an adolescent group indicates that both English and Spanish were frequently used during group sessions (Delgado and Siff, 1980).

PARTICIPANT CHARACTERISTICS

When the Hispanic origin of participants is indicated, Puerto Ricans are the most frequently mentioned group (Delgado and Siff, 1980; Franklin and Kaufman, 1982; Hardy-Fanta and Montana, 1982; Menikoff, 1979; Normand, Iglesias, and Payn, 1974; Rodriguez, 1971; Tylim, 1982), followed by Mexicans (Acosta, 1982; Herrera and Sanchez, 1976; Hynes and Werbin, 1977; Kogeler and

Williamson, 1973; Maduro, 1976; Werbin and Hynes, 1975). Cubans were part of four groups (Acosta, 1982; Delgado and Siff, 1980; Franklin and Kaufman, 1982; Tylim, 1982). Colombians (Franklin and Kaufman, 1982; Tylim, 1982), Nicaraguans (Hynes and Werbin, 1975; Werbin and Hynes, 1975), El Salvadorians (Hynes and Werbin, 1977; Werbin and Hynes, 1975), Panamanians (Werbin and Hynes, 1975) are also specifically mentioned. Finally, Central Americans of an unspecified country of origin were part of three groups (Acosta, 1982; Hardy-Fanta and Montana, 1982; Koegler and Williamson, 1973).

Group composition could be either homogeneous or heterogeneous in terms of Hispanic backgrounds of participants. In examining this, an interesting pattern emerges. Homogeneous groups were composed of Mexicans (Herrera and Sanchez, 1976; Maduro, 1976) and Puerto Ricans (Menikoff, 1979; Normand, Iglesias, and Payn, 1974; Rodriguez, 1971). However, the largest category involves the combination of two or more Hispanic groups. Puerto Ricans were likely to be combined with other groups, i.e., with Cubans (Delgado and Siff, 1980) and other Caribbeans and Central and South Americans (Cooper and Hernandez-Cento, 1977; Hynes and Werbin, 1977; Koegler and Williamson, 1973; Werbin and Hynes, 1975).

Eight articles are based upon female groups (Delgado and Siff, 1980; Hardy-Fanta and Montana, 1982; Franklin and Kaufman, 1982; Hynes and Werbin, 1977; Kraidman, 1980; Leon, 1981; Menikoff, 1979; Werbin and Hynes, 1975) and one upon a male group (Rodriguez, 1971). Additionally, six articles describe group efforts with male and female participants (Acosta, 1982; Herrera and Sanchez, 1976; Koegler and Williamson, 1973; Maduro, 1976; Normand, Iglesias, and Payn, 1974; Tylim, 1982) and one article does not specify sex of participants.

In articles reporting age of group participants, three focus on children and youth ages 11 to 16 (Delgado and Siff, 1980; Hardy-Fanta and Montana, 1982; Richmond et al., 1977), three on 30- to 60-year-olds (Hynes and Werbin, 1977; Kraidman, 1980; Menikoff, 1979), and one on 60- to 72-year-olds (Franklin and Kaufman, 1982). The remaining five articles concern groups that served a very wide range in ages—teens through 40s (Cooper and Hernandez-Cento, 1977), teens through 50s (Herrera and Sanchez, 1976), teens through 70s (Koegler and Williamson, 1973; Tylim, 1982), and 20s to 70s (Werbin and Hynes, 1975).

LEADER CHARACTERISTICS

Groups led by one leader were almost evenly divided between males (Acosta, 1982; Maduro, 1976; Normand, Iglesias, and Payn, 1974; Rodriguez, 1971) and females (Cooper and Hernandez-Cento, 1977; Franklin and Kaufman, 1982; Kraidman, 1980; Menikoff, 1979). Groups with two leaders generally combined a male and female leader (Delgado and Siff, 1980; Hynes and Werbin, 1977; Koegler and Williamson, 1973; Tylim, 1982; Werbin and Hynes, 1975). Female co-leaders (Hardy-Fanta and Montana, 1982) as well as male co-leaders (Herrera and Sanchez, 1976) were also used.

Five articles involve co-leadership by an Hispanic and non-Hispanic (Delgado and Siff, 1980; Hardy-Fanta and Montana, 1982; Hynes and Werbin, 1977; Koegler and Williamson, 1973; Werbin and Hynes, 1975). Six entail one Hispanic leader (Acosta, 1982; Cooper and Hernandez-Cento, 1977; Leon, 1981; Maduro, 1976; Normand, Iglesias, and Payn, 1974; Rodriguez, 1971), three a non-Hispanic leader (Franklin and Kaufman, 1982; Kraidman, 1980; Menikoff, 1979) and two report Hispanic co-leaders (Herrera and Sanchez, 1976; Tylim, 1982).

In examining the particular Hispanic origin of the leaders, Mexicans were the most represented (Acosta, 1982; Herrera and Sanchez, 1976; Maduro, 1976), followed by Puerto Ricans (Delgado and Siff, 1980; Koegler and Williamson, 1973), and Cubans (Hynes and Werbin, 1977; Werbin and Hynes, 1975); there was also one Argentinian (Tylim, 1982).

PRACTICE ISSUES

Practice issues are identified in both empirical and theoretical literature, the bases for the review below. Issues covered include: (1) recruitment, (2) interpersonal group themes, (3) environmental group themes, (4) activities, and (5) possible facilitating factors.

Recruitment

With the exception of two articles (Richmond et al., 1977; Rodriguez, 1971), the source of group recruitment was multiple in nature. Mental health professionals (psychiatrists, psychiatric nurses, and social workers) were the most frequent referral sources (Cooper and Hernandez-Cento, 1977; Franklin and Kaufman, 1982; Hynes and Werbin, 1977; Koegler and Williamson, 1973; Kraidman, 1980; Maduro, 1976; Werbin and Hynes, 1975), followed by social or community agencies (Brown, 1981; Kraidman, 1980; Werbin and Hynes, 1975), school personnel (Brown, 1981; Delgado and Siff, 1980; Hardy-Fanta and Montana, 1982), and the courts (Kraidman, 1980; Richmond et al., 1977).

Some authors note the importance of having a previous relationship with group members before formation of the group (Brown, 1981; Delgado, forthcoming; Delgado and Siff, 1980; Hardy-Fanta and Montana, 1982; Hynes and Werbin, 1977). The importance of interviewing prospective group members also emerges as an aspect in the recruitment process (Cooper and Hernandez-Cento, 1977; Delgado and Siff, 1980; Hardy-Fanta and Montana, 1982; Tylim, 1982).

Interpersonal Group Themes

The literature is replete with interpersonal themes that have particular importance to Hispanics. The most frequently mentioned theme is cultural, marital, and familial conflicts (Acosta, 1982; Delgado and Siff, 1980; Franklin and Kaufman, 1982; Hardy-Fanta and Montana, 1982; Herrera and Sanchez, 1976; Hynes and Werbin, 1977; Kraidman, 1980; Martinez, 1977; Menikoff, 1979; Normand, Iglesias, and Payn, 1974; Rodriguez, 1971; Werbin and Hynes, 1975). Loneliness, as evidenced by personal losses of family members and uprootment from country of origin, is also a prevalent theme (Delgado, 1983, forthcoming; Franklin and Kaufman, 1982; Hardy-Fanta and Montana, 1982; Hynes and Werbin, 1977; Maduro, 1976; Normand, Iglesias, and Payn, 1974; Rodriguez, 1971), along with depression (Delgado, 1983, forthcoming; Herrera and Sanchez, 1976; Normand, Iglesias & Payn, 1974; Menikoff, 1979).

A different set of themes, but nonetheless very popular, focuses on physical health conditions (Franklin and Kaufman, 1982; Kraidman, 1980; Menikoff, 1979), and somatic complaints (Acosta, 1982; Boulette, 1975; Delgado, 1983, forthcoming; Franklin and Kaufman, 1982; Herrera and Sanchez, 1976; Hynes and Werbin, 1977; Normand, Iglesias, and Payn, 1974; Tylim, 1982; Werbin and Hynes, 1975).

The need for social supports within and without the group appears in five articles (Delgado, 1983, forthcoming; Delgado and Siff, 1980; Leon, 1981; Leon, et al., 1981). Violence and fighting (Brown, 1981; Delgado and Siff, 1980; Hardy-Fanta and Montana, 1982; Richmond et al., 1977), a need for a positive self-esteem (Delgado and Siff, 1980; Leon, 1981; Leon et al., 1977), drug and alcohol abuse (Kraidman, 1980; Normand, Iglesias, and Payn, 1974; Rodriguez, 1971), and passivity or fatalism (Delgado, forthcoming; Kraidman, 1980; Werbin and Hynes, 1975) are also mentioned in the literature.

Environmental Group Themes

Environmental group themes are not mentioned as frequently in the literature as interpersonal themes. Nevertheless, two themes are very prevalent—understanding or seeking human services (Delgado, forthcoming; Delgado and Siff, 1980; Koegler and Williamson, 1973; Kraidman, 1980; Leon, 1981; Menikoff, 1979; Normand, Iglesias, and Payn, 1974; Rodriguez, 1971) and the impact of discrimination (Acosta, 1982; Boulette, 1975; Delgado, 1983, forthcoming; Delgado and Siff, 1980; Herrera and Sanchez, 1976). The following themes are also cited in the literature: economic hardships (Delgado, 1983, forthcoming; Martinez, 1977), unemployment (Boulette, 1975), lack of education (Boulette, 1975; Brown, 1981; Hardy-Fanta and Montana, 1982; Normand, Iglesias, and Payn, 1974), and the need to exercise control over the environment (Delgado, 1983; Leon, 1981).

Activities

The literature makes reference to countless numbers of activities that have proved useful in working with Hispanics. Field trips to recreational facilities and community agencies are often cited (Delgado, 1983; Delgado and Siff, 1980; Hynes and Werbin, 1977; Rodriguez, 1971). The use of role play and modeling also emerge as significant (Boulette, 1975; Delgado and Siff, 1980; Herrera and Sanchez, 1976; Kraidman, 1980). Other activities mentioned include: presentation of family history (Delgado, 1983), bringing and eating food (Delgado, 1983; Werbin and Hynes, 1975), yoga exercises (Hynes and Werbin, 1977), parties (Hynes and Werbin, 1977), and invitational lectures (Cooper and Hernandez-Cento, 1977).

Possible Facilitating Factors

Several possible facilitating factors for successful groups with Hispanics emerge from a review of the literature. Half the articles make reference to utilizing contacts with, or at least being aware of, members' contacts with "natural support systems" (Delgado and Humm-Delgado, 1982) such as indigenous healers or family members (Brown and Arevalo, 1979; Cooper and Hernandez-Cento, 1977; Delgado, 1981, 1983, forthcoming; Herrera and Sanchez, 1976; Hynes and Werbin, 1977; Koegler and Williamson, 1973; Kraidman, 1980; Martinez, 1977; Richmond et al., 1977; Rodriguez, 1971; Tylim, 1982; Werbin and Hynes, 1975). This can range from the leader meeting members' families to being accepting of members' contacts with spiritists.

Not surprisingly, the importance of language is also often noted (Boulette, 1975; Herrera and Sanchez, 1976; Delgado, 1981, forthcoming; Martinez, 1977; Normand, Iglesias, and Payn, 1974; Rodriguez, 1971; Ruiz, 1975; Tylim, 1982). This covers factors such as how the use of Spanish fosters group cohesion and how bilingualism can allow flexibility in members expressing themselves.

The need for an action orientation with a focus on the present, rather than past or future, is frequently recommended (Boulette, 1975; Delgado, 1981, 1983; Hynes and Werbin, 1977; Kraidman, 1980; Normand, Iglesias, and Payn, 1974). To facilitate this, many authors suggest the use of structured activities (Boulette, 1975; Brown, 1981; Cooper and Hernandez-Cento, 1977; Delgado, 1983, forthcoming; Delgado and Siff, 1980; Herrera and Sanchez, 1976; Hynes and Werbin, 1977; Kraidman, 1980; and Rodriguez, 1971). Activities supplement a strickly talk-oriented approach so common in traditional group psychotherapy.

The need for sensitivity to Hispanic culture by the leader is stressed by several articles (Delgado, 1981, forthcoming; Koegler and Williamson, 1973; Martinez, 1977; Ruiz, 1975; Tylim, 1982; Werbin and Hynes, 1975). The specific cultural background of the leader is also seen as a facilitating factor for group success by some authors (Delgado and Siff, 1980; Herrera and Sanchez, 1976; Tylim, 1982). The leader may be of the same Hispanic background as group members, of Hispanic background but from a different country of origin than members, or a non-Hispanic co-leader; however, all require knowledge of the particular group members' cultures. In addition, it is suggested that leaders examine their counter-transference towards members as it relates to cultural issues (Leon et al., 1981; Menikoff, 1979; Tylim, 1982).

It is often stated that successful groups tend to be those that operate in a cooperative rather than a competitive or confrontational manner (Acosta, 1982; Delgado, 1983; Hynes and Werbin, 1977; Jimenez, 1981; Normand, Iglesias, and Payn, 1974; Ruiz, 1975). This atmosphere allows for expression of cultural values such as dignity ("dignidad"), respect ("respecto"), and honor ("honor"). Another cultural value that the literature suggests is that group leaders must understand is "personalismo," a tendency to relate to individuals per se rather than institutions (Cooper and Hernandez-Cento, 1977; Delgado, 1983, forthcoming; Leon et al., 1981).

A socialization period before and after the actual group meeting time is also recommended (Delgado, 1983, forthcoming; Delgado and Siff, 1980; Werbin and Hynes, 1975), and leaders have to plan time and space for this. It can also be useful to group process to encourage member contact outside scheduled group times (Cooper and Hernandez-Cento, 1977; Delgado and Siff, 1980; Kraidman, 1980).

Other facilitators for starting or maintaining groups suggested in the literature include such logistical factors as provision of transportation (Delgado, 1981, 1983, forthcoming; Hynes and Werbin, 1977; Werbin and Hynes, 1975), solving child care problems of members during the group session time (Hynes and Werbin, 1977), and using simple intake procedures (Delgado, forthcoming). The use of a short-term group contract is also seen as a facilitating factor by some authors (Delgado, forthcoming; Delgado and Siff, 1980; Hardy-Fanta and Montana, 1982).

Other suggestions for group leaders include: develop a homogeneous group composition in terms of culture, problems, and ages (Franklin and Kaufman, 1982); utilize humor in group discussions (Boulette, 1975); avoid a focus on mental illness (Delgado, forthcoming); and, when appropriate, share one's own experiences, thoughts, and feelings in discussion (Delgado, 1983). The use of dreams for exploration of cultural roots was also found useful (Maduro, 1976).

CONCLUSION

Group work with Hispanics of varying ages and countries of origin has been reported in the literature to be successful in a variety of settings, most often outpatient mental health settings. Additionally, although specific acculturation levels of group members is not generally reported, there appears to be some range in this, e.g., older Hispanics primarily Spanish-speaking versus adolescents comfortable in both English and Spanish.

In forming and conducting groups with Hispanics, it is obvious that certain considerations should be kept in mind. Differences within the Hispanic culture should be acknowledged and understood, since it appears that Hispanics from different countries of origin are often combined within groups. Hispanics of widely varying age ranges are also often combined, but it would seem that this may create more of a communication gap than different Hispanic subgroups would in terms of factors such as language choice and experience on the mainland versus the country of origin. One wonders if the combination of widely varying ages is a function of the small number of Hispanics in a particular agency at a particular time, i.e., the need to combine sufficient people to form a group. While understandable, this combination should probably be carefully evaluated when the range includes adolescents with much older adults. Acculturation levels, too, should probably be assessed at group formation, and a determination made as to whether to mix levels or keep the level rather homogeneous within the group.

Both short-term and long-term groups are reported to be successful. However, in many instances it seems that even the long-term model does not follow a traditional group psychoanalytic model. Differences for which the leader should no doubt strive include the use of activities; focus on problem-solving in the here and now; sharing of one's own thoughts and feelings at times; encouraging contact among members before and after meetings and outside the group sessions; and encouraging a comfortable, cooperative atmosphere that upholds Hispanic cultural values. Additionally, it should be emphasized that recruitment may often be unsuccessful if the leader does not take the necessary amount of time to get to know prospective individual members. It may also be necessary to be willing to establish some contact with the participants' support systems, e.g., family members.

Many interpersonal themes may not in fact be very different from those in any group, e.g., depression. However, others may be more unique to Hispanics, such as somatic complaints. The latter should be expected and accepted in that it is culturally acceptable to express life problems in physical terms; conversely, "mental illness" is not a culturally acceptable designation of a response to a problem.

Another theme that is likely to be found in Hispanic groups more so than other groups is the use of indigenous healers; this, too, should not be viewed automatically as "mental illness" by the leader, since it is so prevalent within the culture. While someone who consults a healer may indeed have emotional problems, the act of consulting the healer should not be cause for labeling the person automatically.

Environmental themes such as economic problems may be more a function of income level than ethnicity, with the exception of certain forms of discrimination. More than talk may be necessary to deal with environmental problems, and so the leader may have to become a broker of concrete services for members at times.

Finally, although settings other than mental health ones are not very evident in the literature, this may be more a function of reporting than actual occurrence. Nevertheless, the use of groups in any setting that serves Hispanics should be encouraged, since the modality, when used in a culturally sensitive way, appears to provide good results for group members.

REFERENCE NOTE

1. The authors have used the following sources for identifying articles that were based on groups and Hispanics: Journals—American Journal of Orthopsychiatry; Group, Hospital & Community Psychiatry; International Journal of Group Psychotherapy; Psychiatric Annals; Psychotherapy: Theory, Research & Practice; Small Group Behavior; Social Work; Social Work in Education; Social Work Research and Abstracts; and Social Work with Groups; Books—reviewed books on Hispanic mental health.

REFERENCES

Acosta, F.K. Group psychotherapy with Spanish speaking patients. In R.M. Becerra, M. Karno, & J.I. Escobar, Eds. *Mental Health and Hispanic Americans: Clinical Perspectives*. New York: Grune and Stratton, 1982.

Boulette, T.R. Group therapy for low-income Mexican Americans. *Social Work*, 1975, *20*, 403-407.

Brown, J.A. Parent education groups for Mexican-Americans. *Social Work in Education*, 1981, *3*, 22-31.

Brown, J.A. and Arevalo, R. Chicanos and social group work models: Some implications for group work practice. *Social Work With Groups*, 1979, *2*, 331-342.

Cooper, E.J. and Hernandez-Cento, M. Group and the Hispanic prenatal patient. *American Journal of Orthopsychiatry*, 1977, 47, 689-700.

Delgado, M. Hispanic cultural values: Implications for groups. *Small Group Behavior*, 1981, *12*, 69-80.

Delgado, M. Activities and Hispanic groups: Issues and recommendations. *Social Work with Groups*, 1983, *6*, 85-96.

Delgado, M. Hispanics and psychotherapeutic groups: Issues and approaches for group leaders. *International Journal of Group Psychotherapy*, forthcoming.

Delgado, M. and Humm-Delgado, D. Natural support systems: Source of strength in Hispanic communities. *Social Work*, 1982, *27*, 83-89.
Delgado, M. and Siff, S. A Hispanic adolescent group in a public school setting: An interagency approach. *Social Work with Groups*, 1980, *3*, 73-85.
Franklin, G.S. and Kaufman, K.S. Group psychotherapy for elderly female Hispanic outpatients. *Hospital and Community Psychiatry*, 1982, *33*, 385-387.
Hardy-Fanta, C. and Montana, P. The Hispanic female adolescent: A group therapy model.
International Journal Of Group Psychotherapy, 1982, *32*, 351-366.
Herrera, A.E. and Sanchez, V.C. Behaviorally oriented group therapy: A successful application in the treatment of low-income Spanish-speaking clients. In M. Miranda, Ed. *Psychotherapy for the Spanish-Speaking*. Los Angeles: Spanish-Speaking Mental Health
Research Center, University of California, 1976.
Hynes, K. and Werbin, J. Group psychotherapy for Spanish-speaking women. *Psychiatric
Annals*, 1977, *7*, 52-63.
Jimenez, D.R. *A comparative analysis of the support systems of White and Puerto Rican
clients in drug treatment programs*. Saratoga, CA: Century Twenty One Publishing,
1980.
Koegler, R.R. and Williamson, E.R. A group approach to helping emotionally disturbed
Spanish-speaking patients. *Hospital and Community Psychiatry*, 1973, *24*, 334-337.
Kraidman, M. Group therapy with Spanish-speaking clinic patients to enhance ego functioning. *Group*, 1980, 4, 59-64.
Leon, A.M. Presentation of a Hispanic mothers support model. In the *First Tri-Regional
Puerto Rican/Hispanic Child Abuse and Neglect Conference*. Trenton, NJ, 1981, 52-54.
Leon, A.M., et al. Self-help support groups for Hispanic parents. In the *First Tri-Regional
Puerto Rican/Hispanic Child Abuse and Neglect Conference*. Trenton, NJ, 1981, 49-51.
Maduro, R. Journey dreams in Latino group psychotherapy. *Psychotherapy: Theory, Research and Practice*, 1976, *13*, 148-155.
Martinez, C. Group process and the Chicano: Clinical issues. *International Journal of Group
Psychotherapy*, 1977, *27*, 225-231.
Menikoff, A. Long-term group psychotherapy of Puerto Rican women: Ethnicity as a clinical
support. *Group*, 1979, *3*, 172-180.
Normand, W.C., Iglesias, J., and Payn, S. Brief group therapy to facilitate utilization of
mental health services by Spanish-speaking patients. *American Journal of Orthopsychiatry*, 1974, *44*, 37-42.
Richmond, A.H., et al. Day treatment of Hispanic adolescents involved with the courts. In
E.R. Padilla and A.M. Padilla, Eds. *Transcultural Psychiatry: An Hispanic Perspective*.
Los Angeles: Spanish-Speaking Mental Health Research Center, University of California, 1977.
Rodriguez, I.D. Group work with hospitalized Puerto Rican patients. *Hospital and Community Psychiatry*, 1971, *22*, 219-220.
Ruiz, E.J. Influence of bilingualism on communication in groups. *International Journal
of Group Psychotherapy*, 1975, *25*, 391-395.
Ruiz, P. Synposium: Group therapy with minority group patients introduction. *International
Journal of Group Psychotherapy*, 1975, *25*, 389-390.
Tylim, I. Group psychotherapy with Hispanic patients: The psychodynamics of idealization. *International Journal of Group Psychotherapy*, 1982, *32*, 339-350.
Werbin, J. and Hynes, K. Transference and culture in a Latino group. *International Journal
of Group Psychotherapy*, 1975, *25*, 396-401.

Essential Components of Group Work with Black Americans

Larry E. Davis

ABSTRACT. The article addresses what the author believes to be some of the fundamentals of group work with Black Americans. Three areas of concern are given priority: knowledge of Black Americans, knowledge of group dynamics pertinent to conducting groups which contain one or more black members, and the importance of employing group work models which have a strong person-environment focus. The article is written from a "before you practice group work with Black Americans" perspective. It is addressed principally to black and white group practitioners, who lead either racially homogeneous or heterogeneous groups.

INTRODUCTION

Despite a wealth of social work literature attesting to the significance of race in the therapeutic encounter, most practitioners who begin group practice with Black Americans are probably ill prepared to do so. There is perhaps no topic of discussion which takes place in a black-white gathering of any sort that heightens anxiety levels more so than a discussion of race itself; indeed, even when not introduced, race is an issue. Therefore, as a preface to the following pages, let us begin by stating that race as an issue is always a salient interpersonal factor and, hence, always has significance for both group members and leaders. With this as our perspective, we will outline and discuss what we believe to be some of the essential components of group work with black Americans. The information presented is not to be viewed as a substitute for a sound and basic training in group work skills; rather it is to be employed as

Larry E. Davis is Associate Professor of Social Work and Psychology, The George Warren Brown School of Social Work, Washington University, St. Louis, Missouri.

97

an integral part of that training. And although the focus of our attentions here will be limited to blacks and whites, we believe that many of the issues addressed have potential relevance for all practitioners of all colors who work with blacks in groups. Moreover, given that most individuals who practice group work are white, while many who are recipients of that treatment are black, the occurrence of racially heterogeneous groups is likely to be, and remain, common place. Hence, we have elected to focus considerable attention upon the white worker who is currently leading groups or contemplating beginning a group which contains black members. However, black group leaders should also benefit significantly from this discussion as it addresses issues which are pertinent to their leadership of both racially homogeneous and heterogeneous groups.

KNOWLEDGE OF BLACK AMERICANS

As a first step in working with blacks, we recommend that group leaders become familiar with blacks as a unique American minority group. They should know that historically, blacks have been isolated from mainstream America. Blacks have not, as a group, elected to separate themselves apart from white America; instead, they have been segregated from it. They were at first segregated as slaves and later as second class citizens. Segregation was, until the 1950s, the law of the land. Today it is less the law, but still the rule. Perhaps Booker T. Washington's statement on black-white social relations best captures America's interracial history as it pertains to blacks, "In all things purely social we can be as separate as the fingers (on the hand)," (Washington, 1895). And despite the attempts of many individuals and organizations, socially America remains a society largely partitioned by color. Such partitioning has left both blacks and whites suspicious, unfamiliar, and consequently, more often than not, uncomfortable when in the other's presence.

Due to the extent of racial segregation and because of the greater numbers of whites than blacks, whites often have little personal experience with, or knowledge of, Black Americans. Indeed, whites may suffer from both a lack of information and/or misinformation pertaining to blacks. In an effort to correct this situation, we recommend that practitioners be exposed to positive educational materials on Black Americans. Such exposure and education may provide a corrective and informative experience. It is beyond the scope of this paper to provide the needed information in sufficient detail. However, there are several books on this subject that should aid group leaders in obtaining a rudimentary understanding of Black Americans. Two such texts are *From Slavery to Freedom*, by J. Franklin (1969), and *Blacks in White America Since 1865*, by R. Twombly (1971). Either of these books will afford group leaders a historical perspective beneficial to their work with Black clients.

In addition to a sound understanding of blacks as a people, those who work therapeutically with black Americans should also have some knowledge of blacks as a treatment population. There exists at this time a great deal of theoretical and empirical literature which addresses the salience of race in the therapeutic relationship (Beckett, 1980; Banks, 1971; Goodman, 1969; Sue, 1977, 1981; Dana, 1981; Green, 1982). Clearly there exists less literature which specifically addresses group work with Black Americans. However, there does exist a sufficient number of articles to negate the perennial statement that "good literature on this topic cannot be found" (Brayboy, 1971, 1974; Cobbs, 1972; Davis, 1979, 1981). Unfortunately, however, the client outcome literature on group work with blacks still needs greater specificity with regards to the explicit treatment interventions and modalities employed. Additionally, greater attention must be paid to actual client outcomes rather than to client evaluations of the group experience. Specific to our purpose here, it is important that practitioners know that blacks do not use mental health services as extensively as do whites, have higher attrition rates, and are more often referred to group forms of treatment (Sattler, 1977); and that blacks often prefer black professionals over white professionals (Banks, 1972; Brieland, 1969; Carkhuff and Pierce, 1967). On the other side of the coin, group workers should know that practitioner ethnocentrism is negatively related to the selection of non-whites as clients (Yamamoto, James, Bloombaum, and Hattern, 1967) and that there is some evidence to suggest that practitioners feel more appropriately responsive to same race clients, (Fry, Kopf, and Coe, 1980).

KNOWLEDGE OF RACIAL DYNAMICS

As a consequence of America's peculiar minority-majority group history, black-white and even black-black interactions present a unique challenge to group leaders. Hence, in addition to possessing knowledge about blacks as a people, it is also useful for practitioners to be cognizant of how race may affect the dynamics of group treatment. We shall provide an essential introduction to some of the most common and salient racial dynamics which confront members and leaders of either homogeneous or heterogeneous racial groups. Specifically, we shall inspect the following as they affect group dynamics: group composition, race as an issue, the absence of trust, and member statuses and roles.

Group Composition

The law of attraction (Byrne, 1971) suggests that individuals who are similar to one another should be most attracted to each other. Hence, we might conjecture that a group composition consisting of all blacks should experience fewer difficulties than a racialy mixed group. In general, this assertion is probably correct. However, groups consisting of all blacks may also experience difficulties which can be attributed to the groups racial composition.

In a candid discussion of group experiences in an all black treatment group, Davis, Sharfstein, and Owens (1974) poignantly identified a number of potential problems. They indicated that although treatment experiences with an all-black group composition resulted in an overall positive experience for the members, the group was not without some unique problems. The authors reported that members of their newly formed group questioned the legitimacy of an all-black group. Some members questioned if the treatment experience would be ''legitimate therapy,'' or if members would only talk about their blackness and not their problems. Their concern was that treatment might be compromised in the absence of white group members. Davis et al. indicated that such concerns, after a period of time, dissipated.

A second problem which Davis and his colleagues outlined had to do with the group's leader being black. As some members had questioned a black group's legitimacy, some members questioned the black leader's legitimacy. That is, some members queried the leader as to his competency to lead a group. Specifically, they expressed doubts about his therapeutic training and abilities. In time, this challenge was also overcome and the leader went on to lead a successful group; however, it did give the group leader cause for concern. The treatment group described by Davis et al. (1974) took place in the early 1970s and, hence, we might expect that due to the social, political, and educational advances which blacks have made since that time, fewer clients are likely to receive an all-black group or a group led by a black with such reservations. However, even today it would be safe to assume that, although some clients would welcome and enjoy an opportunity to be in an all black group, others may view such a group as lacking legitimacy and their inclusion in it a form of segregation. In this same view, the black leader of all black groups, more so than the black leader of a racially mixed group, may be more open to questions of legitimacy as the members may ponder why he or she was not assigned or "allowed" to treat whites also.

The black leader is not alone in challenges to his leadership. White leaders may also receive challenges from black group members. There is some evidence that the degree of "militancy" of black clients is negatively associated with the acceptance of the white therapist (Sattler, 1977). Hence, the white group leader may be resisted or challenged not only because he is perceived as being insufficiently skilled or knowledgeable to help blacks, but also because black clients may be reluctant for political or philosophical reasons to accept white leadership.

Problems revolving around group composition are not limited to the racially homogeneous black group. The thoroughness of America's racial separation has mitigated significantly meaningful interactions between blacks and whites. It is due to this legacy of restricted black-white contact that the issue of the heterogeneous group composition takes on such unique importance. Even today, interactions that do occur between blacks and whites are largely limited to perfunctory and superficial encounters. As a result, most whites, and many blacks also, may experience their first "quality" contact with racially dissimilar others in groups which were created for therapeutic purposes. However, because of their minority numbers and status, blacks as a group frequently have had more exposure and contact with whites than whites have had with blacks. Consequently, black-white interactions are more likely to be anxiety arousing experiences for whites than for blacks (Davis, 1975). This phenomenon is likely to be true for both leaders and members. That is, it is probable that white leaders, as well as white members, may experience more anxiety in racially mixed groups than will the blacks in those groups. As a result, the beginning phase of the racially heterogeneous treatment group may be even more anxiety-arousing than are the beginnings of most groups. Therefore, the group leader's initial behaviors and reactions are of great significance to the racially heterogeneous group. Indeed, whether the leader is black or white, his initial contact with the group will establish the tone of future contact and to a great extent determine if the group members will establish positive and sincere contact with each other (Newcomb, 1947; Mizio, 1972). In light of this, an important first objective of the leader of a racially heterogeneous group is to make the initial group meetings as pleasant and as non-anxiety-arousing as possible.

The specific racial ratio of an integrated group may also be a significant and important issue to the group's leader and members. There has been some attention given to this issue in the literature (Brayboy, 1974; Winter, 1971; Davis, 1979). Surprisingly, however, many group work texts have had little, if anything, to say regarding the implications of a group's racial composition (Glasser, Sarri, and Vinter, 1974; Garvin, 1981; Konopka, 1983). Despite this often overlooked topic, the issue of how many blacks and whites to include in a particular group is sometimes an important decision which the group leader must make.

How many blacks and whites should be in any particular group? Attempting to answer this question is perhaps one of the factors which makes working with racially heterogeneous groups uniquely difficult. Indeed, some research indicates that blacks and whites may have different conceptions of what the racial balance of small groups ought to be (Davis 1979). Blacks, it appears, prefer groups that are 50 percent black and 50 percent white—numerical equality. Whites, on the other hand, appear to prefer groups that are approximately 20 percent black and 80 percent white, societal ratios of blacks and whites. Needless to say, the preferences of both groups cannot be simultaneously met. This difference in preference for racial balance has the potential to lead to member dissatisfaction, discomfort, and withdrawal. For example, it has been witnessed that whites may be reluctant to become members of groups in which they are a minority (Brayboy, 1974). Davis (1980) contends that white reluctance to be in the minority has to do with a state of psychological balance. He posits that whites, because of their customary numerical dominance, feel themselves to be psychologically in the minority or outnumbered, if blacks are present in numbers greater than their societal proportions. Moreover, there are indications that some group practitioners are reticent to introduce even a single black into their treatment groups (Rosenbaum and Hartley, 1966).

Finally, it should also be noted that the salience of a group member's race appears to increase as the intimacy of the group increases (Triandis and Davis, 1965; Davis, 1979). That is, as the probability of group intimacy increases either because of the group's task topic or size, the racial identities of the other group members included in the group is likely to increase in importance. Therefore, it would seem prudent, when and if possible, to always include at least two members of each racial group if the group is to be an intimate one. Such inclusions should serve potentially to prevent tokenism, reduce the probability of scapegoating, and provide each member with a "second opinion" by which to more accurately assess his/her perception of social reality.

Acknowledging the Salience of Race

It is advisable that the leader, whether black or white, promote in the very early stages of group formation a discussion of the group's racial composition. Such a discussion may afford individuals an opportunity to express any concerns which they might have. A discussion of the group's racial composition will also serve the very valuable purpose of both introducing the topic and acknowledging the salience of race. While there probably exists no best way to introduce this highly affect-laden issue, it is an issue which should not be avoided if the black members are to have open and honest discussions. Because race has played such a significant role in the lives of blacks, it is generally a topic of considerable importance to them. It has been sometimes noted that, in racially heterogeneous groups of blacks and whites, blacks try to point out the salience of race as a factor affecting life events, while whites may simultaneous attempt to deny its influence (Brayboy, 1971). If it occurs, this phenomenon should be acknowledged and its implications for the group discussed.

On the other hand, the leader should not be surprised if his efforts to introduce race as an issue are met with some initial resistance. Race is a topic laden with a great deal of affect. Consequently, both blacks and whites may, as a matter of practice, attempt to circumvent a racial discussion. Here again, we wish to emphasize that race is always salient, and to feign color blindness does a great disservice to the group process by relegating group member interactions to a superficial level. Group leaders of biracial groups are often afraid to introduce race as a topic for group discussion for fear of heightening or creating racial tension. Certainly there is some risk, but there is a greater probability of relieving group tension by openly acknowledging what all are already thinking. By doing so, the group leader sanctions future discussions of race. In other words, he says to the group members that it's "OK" to discuss race. Introducing race as a topic for discussion also models honesty to the group members, in that the leader is not pretending to be oblivious to a very obvious and salient descriptive attribute of each member. Hence, despite possible group member resistance, and leader apprehension at the introduction of race as an issue, its introduction will provide a valuable service to the group.

Coping with the Absence of Trust

If the practitioner is to establish a viable relationship with the group members, he/she must somehow manage to establish a basis of trust. Unfortunately, the sociopolitical history of blacks in America has been one riddled with their betrayal. Hence, it is not surprising to find an all black or mixed group climate which is characterized by distrust of the sponsoring agency and it representative, the group leader. The consequence of such group member distrust may manifest itself by the occurrence of group member attrition, lack of indepth disclosure, and low rates of member participation.

The source of distrust which black clients may exhibit when in group treatment may be a function of one or both of the following factors: First, they may question the good will of the group members and leader. That is, they may be uncertain as to whether the group members and/or the leader has their best interests at heart. Secondly, they may perceive the non-black members or leader, and possibly even some blacks, as possessing insufficient knowledge of the social realities of black people. In other words, they may view the helper(s) as lacking sufficient understanding of their concerns.

There are no "pat" strategies as to how to hasten the development of trust or desolve distrust which frequently exists between black group members and those trying to help them. Some of these apprehensions will probably fade with time, if the black client remains in the group long enough! However, it is incumbent upon those group workers who work with blacks to be cognizant of the fact that trust may be in short supply—especially in the early phases of group development—and to consequently be patient in their efforts to secure it. Group leaders of interracial groups in particular should periodically ask themselves, what am I or the group members doing to affect the group dynamics so as to encourage or dissuade the development of trust within the group?

Status and Roles

There is literature which suggests that blacks may behave differently in groups depending upon whether the groups are racially heterogeneous or homogeneous (Katz and Benjamin, 1960; Katz and Greenbaum, 1963; Lefcourt and Ladwig, 1965). Sometimes blacks, when in racially mixed groups, have been witnessed to defer leadership and to participate in the group process to a lesser extent than might be expected. Some of this reserved participation may be attributable to a general lack of trust or to, what some have referred to, as healthy paranoia (Grier and Cobbs, 1968). However, some lack of participation on the part of blacks in groups may be attributable to the low social status ascribed to them. As noted earlier, blacks have historically occupied a subordinate social status in America and, as a result, have frequently been limited to subordinate roles. Albeit, black political and social advances have expanded considerably what most believe to be a "black's place," many individuals still hold limited expectations of the roles which blacks should or are capable of playing. Such limited expectations, on the behalf of group members or leaders, may result in a misperception of black behavior. For example, equal participation by blacks may be perceived erroneously as arrogant or aggressive behavior (Cheek, 1976). Correspondingly, some individuals may attempt to thwart the active participation of black group members in an effort to retain them in subordinate roles, while others may ignore their contributions believing them to be unimportant or insignificant to the group process. Needless to say, such low status role conscriptions on black involvement and participation adversely affects black participation in small groups. Not only does it alienate those black members who are ascribed to an inferior role, but it also retards group development by limiting group cohesion and trust, not to mention depriving the group of valuable insight and ideas.

Hence, leaders of groups which have black members should remain alert to the possible occurrence of this racially fostered dynamic. They should remain vigilant in their efforts to see that the attempts of black group members to participate in the group process is neither thwarted nor ignored. It might be a good idea for the leaders of racially heterogeneous groups to periodically assess the approximate participation rate of each member.

A PERSON-ENVIRONMENTAL PERSPECTIVE

Is there a "best" model of group work practice for black clients? There is no evidence to support such a claim. Surely, the absence of such evidence is in part due to the reality that blacks, like other ethnic or racial groups, are not attitudinally or behaviorally a homogeneous collection of individuals who all share the same problem. However, despite the great diversity which exists among blacks— e.g., social economic status, regional identities, etc.—they do share some very important things in common. Among the most important, they perceive themselves and are perceived by society as a distinct racial group. This badge of color, as it is sometimes referred to, results in their perceiving themselves to share a common experience and perhaps a common fate. Frequently their experiences are infused with undeniable and unyielding acts of discrimination, contributing to feelings of oppression and powerlessness. There is, in both the research and practice literature, evidence which suggests that blacks, more so than whites, perceive a great deal of what happens to them as being outside of their personal control and a function of environmental forces (Lefcourt, 1965; Lessing, 1969; Duke and Lewis, 1979). Such perceptions by blacks argue strongly for the employment of a group practice model which incorporates a significant environmental focus into its theoretical formulations.

Although social group work has been slow in adequately addressing race as a practice issue, it continues to recognize the importance of the environment (Garvin, 1981; Balgopal 1983). As does Garvin (1981), we too concur with Robert Vinter that, "All behavior amenable to change is regarded as socially induced, acquired through learning and related processes; it is exhibited, or constrained, within the context of specific social situations. We also concur that the sources of behavior lie both within the *individual* (in terms of his enduring attributes and acquired capabilities) and within the *social situation* (in terms of opportunities, domains, and inducements" (Vinter, 1974-A, p. 4-5).

Such an even-handed conceptualization of individual behavior on the part of the group worker may prove to be especially useful when practicing with blacks whose lives are notably subjected to the influence of factors located within the environment. Hence, we advocate that group leaders who work with blacks adopt an interactional view of client difficulties and, correspondingly, be prepared to engage in environmental interventions, or what have been referred to as extra-group means of influence (Vinter, 1974-B). Thus, in addition to intervening directly or indirectly with members inside the group, the group leader must also be willing to intervene with individuals, groups, or institutions in the client's social environment (Garvin, 1981).

The advocacy here for a strong person-environmental model of group treatment is not to imply that ''black people do not go crazy'' or that all difficulties which they experience can be attributed to environmental factors. Indeed, all groups of individuals, irrespective of ethnicity, experience interpersonal and intrapsychic difficulties. However, we are suggesting that due to the degree and intensity of impact, which the environment is believed to exert on the lives of most black people, any model employed in their treatment which does not have a strong environmental focus is probably incomplete in its conceptualization of their problems and, as a result, probably advocates inadequate intervention strategies.

SUMMARY AND CONCLUSION

This paper has identified three broad areas which are of interest to those practitioners who want to work more effectively with Black Americans in groups. *First*, it argues that all who work with Black Americans should have some rudimentary knowledge of black socio-political history. *Secondly*, the case is made that it is necessary that practitioners have knowledge of the potency which race has on the dynamics of the group, its individual members, and leaders. Specifically, it is suggested that group leaders pay attention to group dynamics as they are effected by a group's racial composition, the salience of race as an issue, the absence of helper-helpee trust, and group member status and roles as possibly influenced by race. And *thirdly*, because blacks are believed to be effected significantly by the social environment, the paper argues for the employment of group work models which have a strong person-environmental focus.

At the risk of overstatement and stereotyping, this article attempts to convey in a few brief pages what the author believes to be some essential information about which practitioners should be cognizant before beginning groups which contain one or more black members. By and large, this article was written from a "before you practice group work with blacks perspective." However, it is intended that even those who have prior group work experience with Black Americans will benefit from reading this paper.

Finally, it is hoped that no one will be displeased by the title of this article which was largely borrowed from a well known contributor to the theory and practice of group work, Robert Vinter (1974-B). As his seminal article, "The Essential Components of Group Work Practice," has aided in the training of a great number of group workers, it is intended that this article will serve as an aid to those being trained to engage in group work with Black Americans.

ESSENTIAL COMPONENTS BIBLIOGRAPHY

Balgopal, P., and Vassil, T., *Groups in social work: An ecological approach.* New York: Macmillan, 1983.

Banks, G., The effects of race on one to one helping interviews. *Social Service Review,* 1971, *45,* 137-146.

Beckett, J., Perspectives on social work intervention and treatment with black clients: A bibliography. *Black Caucus Journal,* 1980, *11,* 24-32.

Brayboy, T., The black patient in group therapy. *International Journal of Group Psychotherapy,* 1971, *21,* 288-293.

Brayboy, T., Black and white groups and therapists. In: D. Milman, and G. Goldman, (eds.). *Group process today: Evaluation and perspective.* Springfield, Ill.: Charles C. Thomas, 1974.

Brieland, D., Black identity and the helping person. *Children,* 1969, *16*(5), 170-176.

Byrne, D., The attraction paradigus. New York: Academic Press, 1971.

Carkhuff, R., and Pierce, R., Differential effects of therapist race and social class upon patient depth of self-exploration in the initial clinical interview. *Journal of Consulting Psychology,* 1967, *31,* 632-634.

Cheek, D., *Assertive black puzzled white: A black perspective on assertive behavior.* California: Impact Publishers, 1976.

Cobbs, P., Ethnotherapy in Groups. In L. Solomon and B. Berzon (eds.). *New Perspectives on Encounter Groups.* San Francisco: Jossey-Bass, Inc., 1972.

Dana, D., *Human services for cultural minorities.* Maryland: Baltimore University Park Press, 1981.

Davis, L., When the majority is the psychological minority. *Group Psychotherapy Psychodrama, and Sociometry,* 1980, *33,* 179-184.

Davis, L., Racial balance: A psychological issue. *Social Work with Groups,* 3(2), 1980, 75-85.

Davis, L., Racial composition of groups. *Social Work,* 1979, *24,* 208-213.

Davis, L., Dynamics of race in therapeutic practice. Unpublished Social Work Doctoral Preliminary Examinations. University of Michigan, 1975.

Davis, M., Sharfstein, S., and Owens, M., Separate and together: All black therapist group in the white hospital. *American Journal of Orthopsychiatry,* 1974, *44,* 19-25.

Duke, M., and Lewis, G., The measurement of locus of control in black preschool and primary school. *Journal of Personality Assessment*, 1979, *43*, 351-355.

Franklin, J., *From slavery to freedom: A history of Negro Americans*. New York: Vintage House, 1969.

Fry, P., Kropf, G., and Coe, K., Effects of counselor and client racial similarity on the counselor's response pattern and skills. *Journal of Consulting Psychology*, 1980, *27*, 130-137.

Garvin, C., *Contemporary group work*. New Jersey: Prentice-Hall, 1981.

Glasser, P., Sarri, R., and Vinter, R., (eds.), *Individual change through small groups*. New York: Free Press, 1974.

Goodman, J. (ed.), *Dynamics of racism in social work practice*. Washington, D.C.: NASW, 1969.

Green, J., *Cultural awareness in the human services*. New Jersey: Prentice-Hall, 1982.

Katz, I., and Benjamin, L., Effects of white authoritarianism is biracial. *Journal of Abnormal and Social Psychology*, 1960, *61*, 448-456.

Katz, I., and Greenbaum, C., Effects of anxiety, threat, and racial environment on task performance of Negro college students. *Journal of Abnormal and Social Psychology*, 1963, *66*, 562-567.

Konopka, G., *Social group work: A helping process*. New Jersey: Prentice Hall, 1983.

Lefcourt, H., and Ladwig, G., The American Negro, problem in expectancies. *Journal of Personality and Social Psychology*, 1965, *1*, 377-380.

Lessing, E., Racial differences in indices of ego functioning relevant to academic achievement. *Journal of Genetic Psychology*, 1969, *115*, 153-167.

Mizio, E., White worker-minority client. *Social Work*, 1972, *17*, 82-86.

Newcomb, T., Autistic hostility and social reality. *Human Relations*, 1947, *1*, 69-87.

Rosenbaum, M., and Hartley, Z., Group psychotherapy and the integration of the Negro. *International Journal of Group Psychotherapy*, 1966, *16*, 86-90.

Sattler, J., The effects of therapist/client similarity. In A. Gurman and A. Razin (Eds.), *Effective psychotherapy: A handbook of research*. New York: Pergamon Press, 1977.

Sue, D., Counseling the culturally different: A conceptual analysis. *Personnel and Guidance Journal*, 1977, *55*, 422-425.

Sue, D., *Counseling the culturally different: Theory and practice*. New York: John Wiley, 1981.

Triandis, H., and Davis, E., Race and belief as determinants of behavioral intentions. *Journal of Personality and Social Psychology*, 1965, *2*, 715-725.

Twombly, R., *Blacks and white America since 1965: Issues and interpretations*. New York: McKay, 1971.

Vinter, R., An approach to group work practice. In P. Glasser, R. Sarri, and R. Vinter (eds.), *Individual change through small groups*. New York: Free Press, 1974-A, 4-5.

Vinter, R., The essential components of group work practice. In P. Glasser, R. Sarri, and R. Vinter, (eds.), *Individual change through small groups*. New York: Free Press, 1974-B, 9-33.

Washington, B., Atlanta Exposition Address. Delivered at the Atlanta Exposition, September 18, 1895.

Winter, S., Black man's bluff. *Psychology Today*, 1971, *5*, 39-43, 78-81.

Yamamoto, J., James, Q., Bloombaum, M., and Hattern, J., Racial factors in patient selection. *American Journal of Psychiatry*, 1967, *124*, 630-636.

Group Work with Low-Income Black Youths

John A. Brown

ABSTRACT. Low-income Black youths face problems which negatively impact on their self-concepts and educational achievement. Without an education, the opportunities for social mobility for them are severely decreased. The small group is suggested as a medium of intervention in the public schools by which large numbers of low-income Black youths can be reached and assisted with problems which interfere with their education. This paper discusses group work with this population, the theoretical framework utilized, and the applicability of some of the insights gained from working with this population to group work with Blacks in general.

This paper discusses group work with low-income Black youths in the public school setting. In addition to identifying and discussing the theoretical framework employed, this paper will present some practice examples as well as identify some of the insights gained from group work with this population and their applicability in working with Blacks in general when the group is employed as the medium of intervention. It is extremely important that effective means of intervention be identified by which large numbers of low-income Black youths can be reached in the public schools and assisted in addressing those problems which impact on them negatively and interfere with their education. The public schools have encountered problems in achieving educational goals with this population (*Challenging the Myths: the Schools, the Blacks and the Poor*, 1973). Equality, the attainment of social justice, the avenues of social mobility, and the emergence of future Black leadership are

John A. Brown is Professor School of Social Work, San Jose State University, San Jose, CA 95192.

111

dependent on educational attainment. The group, by the various purposes it serves, provides an effective medium for intervention into problems faced by large numbers of low-income Black youths in the public schools.

THE SCHOOL SETTING AS ENVIRONMENT FOR PREVENTIVE/HABILITATIVE EFFORTS

American children spend at least 13 years of their lives in a school setting. The school is a major agent of socialization. While a primary responsibility of the school is the education of students for responsible citizenship, public schools can also assume an important role in identifying and addressing problems faced by minority youths. Low-income Black youths have been exposed to institutional, cultural, and psychological racism (Bromley and Longino, 1972). Racist encounters have negatively affected their personality development, self-esteem, and motivation. Their entrance into the public schools is preceded by a social typing, "underachievers," "unmotivated," "culturally deprived"—which literally insures their failure through a self-fulfilling prophecy (Rist, 1973). These youths come to school with social disadvantages which become magnified by the treatment which they encounter within the school. Logan (1981) suggests that "schools have been the place where many Black children's first lesson in self-hate begins reflecting— sometimes conscious, sometimes unconscious—hostility of peers and teachers," (p. 53). Due to the disadvantages which these youths encounter in life in general and the school in particular, the view is expressed here that low-income Black youth are more in need of habilitative than rehabilitative services.

THE CONCEPT OF BLACK SELF-ESTEEM

Inasmuch as these youths have been viewed as inferior persons and live in a society in which they are placed in a non-valued status, they develop negative self-concepts* and face problems with their racial identity. Fisher (1970) states, "The crisis in identity is the

---

*Self-concept as used here refers to a picture which an individual holds of him/herself.

necessity of choosing either dominant group definition or coming to know and appreciate themselves and the contributions they make toward enriching the culture'' (p. 26).

A number of writers (Poussaint and Atkinson, 1973; Banks and Grambs, 1972; Long, 1975) have discussed the self-concepts of low-income Black youths. These youths are viewed as being inferior due to their racial status. As a result of societal experiences, they develop negative views of themselves which become strengthened through their experiences with social institutions. These negative encounters impact adversely on the attitudes of these youths toward the dominant society, their self-concepts, and their abilities. In addition to resolving the crisis of racial identity and in improving their self-concepts, these youths are also called on to resolve the usual crises associated with adolescence. Consequently, the small group above all must provide them with a transforming experience.

OPPORTUNITIES FOR SOCIOPSYCHOLOGICAL DEVELOPMENT AND IMPROVING SELF-CONCEPTS WITHIN THE SMALL GROUP

Group work with low-income Black youths provide an opportunity for the improvement of their self-concepts, the development of improved coping skills, and the validation of racial identification. Group work with these youths, often alienated from American life, requires that the group worker possesses sensitivity to the Black experience. In utilizing the group as an instrument of problem-solving, a vehicle for systems change, and as a medium for strengthening racial validation and improving self-concepts, the group worker must embrace a dual focus on the individual and society and the nature of the interactions and transactions which occur between the two. The group is thus placed at the midway point between these two entities with the group worker assuming an enabling and mediating function. The group worker can never lose sight of the fact that Blacks are viewed by the dominant group as constituting a ''troublesome presence'' and a social problem in American society (Yinger, 1964). The group worker must possess the skills, knowledge, and ability to identify and analyze dysfunctional policies (negative social policies), negative attitudes of school personnel, racist practices and procedures, and the manner by which the school performs and perpetuates the latent function of institutional racism. Low-income Black youths in their interactions and behavior within the group will mirror the effects of societal experiences. The group must provide the opportunity for testing themselves and finding acceptance and validation as they work to develop improved self-concepts and the sociopsychological skills which will enhance their chances for greater success in the public schools.

THEORETICAL FRAMEWORK FOR GROUP INTERVENTION

Low-income Black youths need to be assisted in developing social competencies. Katz (1973) states "some studies indicate that lower-class black children are motivated to gain approval through physical characteristics and process rather than through intellectual achievement as are middle-class white and black children" (Poussaint and Atkinson, 1973, p. 175). Pearson (1968) states,

> Culturally different individuals can be helped to change only if the avenues of change opened to them have some promise of allowing each one to retain his integrity as a person and are perceived as need-satisfying alternatives. (p. 61).

Further, he states, "A relationship. . .in which individuals are accepted and in which he senses that he is considered a person of worth enhances his possibilities for change or development" (p. 61). For low-income Black youths to be motivated to change, they must feel accepted and that the modification in behavior can lead to benefits. They also must feel that the person who is attempting to bring about this change values them as individuals.

Extensive group work literature is not available on group work with Blacks. Considerable literature is available on groups in social work and their use in promoting interpersonal and societal change (Papell and Rothman, 1966; Hartford, 1971; Klein 1972; Glasser, Sarri and Vinter, 1974; Roberts and Northen, 1976 and Shulman, 1979). Some writings are available on group work in particular settings in which Blacks were probably members of the group (*Helping People in Groups,* 1965; *Potentials for Services Through Group Work in Public Welfare,* 1962.) Brayboy (1971) suggests that Blacks have been written about by whites and their views of the Black psyche. For whatever the reason, a void exists in social work literature on group work with Blacks.

Papell and Rothman (1966) identified three models of social group work: social goals, remedial, and reciprocal. The reciprocal model of Schwartz (1977) is also referred to as the interactionist and the mediating model. Generally, the majority of group work approaches can be located under the remedial model in which group efforts are directed toward achieving individual change. As a consequence of the unique position of Blacks in American society and the manner in which social systems impact on them, the reciprocal model of Schwartz has greater utility and applicability for group work with Blacks. Schwartz's model draws on knowledge from social systems and field theory (Whittaker, 1974). Due to its interactionist focus, it also accommodates knowledge from social psychology, particularly role theory and symbolic interactionism. The symbolic interactionism perspective views social selves as developing from a process of interaction with other social selves. Consequently, it offers a useful framework for attempting to modify negative self-concepts through its focus on social selves, how they develop, and the social processes which can modify or maintain self-conceptions (Strauss, 1959; Blumer, 1969).

Key concepts within Schwartz's reciprocal model are symbiotic ties between the individual and society, the group as a mutual-aid system, and the search for a common ground. In this model, the group worker assumes a mediating, enabling role as he/she attempts to address systemic stress. This model has further utility for group work with Blacks as it does not utilize a formal diagnostic process and thus avoids the pitfall of misdiagnosing behavior. Neither does it establish goals for each member. The focus of work emerges from the needs of the group members and the identification of the friction points within the interacting systems. Schwartz's phases of tuning in, contract establishment, work, and termination (Shulman, 1979) provides the means by which the group development over time can be observed and analyzed. In initial contacts, the group worker tunes himself/herself into the needs of the group and it is from the identification of these needs that targets of intervention are identified and activities selected and implemented to bring about change. The group emerges as a task-oriented, problem-solving one in which group members are not viewed as the primary problem-carriers. Inasmuch as low-income Black youths and the school need each other to bring about a functional system, the group worker seeks to identify and locate the common ground in which each has a stake. This approach—locating the common ground when friction occurs between Blacks and interacting systems—is a common and essential element in group work with Blacks in general. In addition to systems and field theory, symbolic interactionism provides strong theoretical underpinnings to this model. It is a theory of human social development which has particular relevance to how negative self-concepts are formed and maintained through a complex system of role behavior. Poussaint and Atkinson (1973) state,

> For the black youth in white American society, the generalized other whose attitudes he assumes and the looking glass self into which he gazes both reflect the same judgement; he is inferior because he is black (p. 168).

Self-concepts can never be separated from the complex environment and the interpersonal relationships from which the person draws his/her sense of self and frame of reference. Since racism is a structural phenomenon with sociopsychological consequences for Blacks, Schwartz's reciprocal model of social group work and the theoretical perspective of symbolic interactionism provide a sound foundation for group work with Blacks, particularly low-income Black youths, in which a primary objective is the improvement of self-concepts.

THE GROUP

John Muir Junior High* provided the setting in which the group discussed in this paper was developed and implemented. This school is located in an urban city of 693,000 containing both urban and rural characteristics. Its location is frequently referred to as the Silicon Valley. This city has a multi-ethnic population and has recently seen a large influx of Vietnamese refugees. The racial/ethnic compositon of John Muir is 1.4 percent Native Americans, 20 percent Pacific Islanders, 16.9 percent Blacks, 32.6 percent Hispanics, and 29.1 others—primarily whites. The socio-economic backgrounds of the students ranged from lower to middle class. The

---

*School is disguised.

majority of the teaching staff were of white middle-class backgrounds. Blacks were a fairly recent introduction to the school and a Black principal also had recently been assigned to John Muir. The principal was concerned over the problems faced by minority youth. The problems faced by these youths included poor grades, negative attitudes toward school, defiance of authority, and suspicion of drugs and truancy. Racial/ethnic confrontations had also occurred. The school's characteristic responses to these youths were to send them to the principal's office or home, expell them from school, or to have them transferred to a special school. Much stress presented itself in teacher-student interactions. It was this concern which led the principal to seek assistance from the local school of social work. Several faculty members met with the principal to discuss the problem, identify how the school could contribute to addressing the problem, and to map strategy. The principal requested specifically that the Black faculty member become involved in the change-process due to the absence of positive role models in the lives of these youths. A similar request was made of the Chicano faculty member (Brown and Arevalo, 1980). The principal also recognized that the low-income Black youths saw him as a member of the establishment.*

The group approach was selected because it provided the opportunity to reach a large number of low-income Black youths in addition to the therapeutic benefits it would provide. It was also consistent with the objectives of intervention: modification of self-concepts, development of social competencies, promoting the growth of sociopsychological skills, and the provision of positive role models with which students might identify and emulate. White social workers, to a degree, may hold certain stereotypes about low-income Black youths which may lead them to engage in victim analysis. They may attempt to change these youths to conform to school expectations instead of identifying and attempting to change the role which the school plays in enforcing and maintaining their behavior. The Black faculty member who became the group worker was familiar with the experiences and needs of these youths. He was a product of a similar background and this fact was beneficial in gaining the group's acceptance.

---

*An interesting dilemma for the Black professional is how he/she is viewed by low-income Black youths. Many times a general suspicion exists that the Black professional has identified with the dominant group, is a part of the establishment, and is not to be trusted.

CHARACTERISTICS AND STRUCTURE OF THE GROUP

Initially, the group was designed as a closed one. Ten low-income Black males identified by school personnel as in need of help formed the original membership. The group quickly evolved by natural development into an open-ended, mixed group due to the interest shown by other Black youths in becoming involved. The group provided them with a sense of importance, something of their own, which set them apart from other students. Before the group, they had literally nothing else in the school with which they could identify. The responsibility of identifying youths who needed the group experience rested with the school. Potential members were referred by teachers to a counselor and subsequently to the group, following discussions with the group worker. The school assumed the responsibility of clearing administrative matters such as securing permission from parents, arranging for students to be released from classes, explaining the purposes of the group to the teaching staff, and enlisting their cooperation. At various times, the group worker met with the principal and the school counselor assigned to the group to discuss its progress and to identify problems. The group was planned to last for a semester and, if possible, to resume the following semester.

In attempting to improve self-concepts and to reconcile, to whatever possible degree, individual stress and system dysfunctioning, the group had to be structured to provide these students with a transforming experience (Strauss, 1969). According to Blumer (1969), "The meaning that things have for human beings are central in their own right and to ignore the meaning of these things toward which people act is seen as falsifying the behavior under study" (p. 7). If low-income Black youths view the school as constituting a negative, uncaring environment and this is reinforced by the experiences and attitudes encountered, then their behavior will reflect such a belief. Consequently, the group worker needs to interface with teachers and administrators in attempting to modify attitudes held toward these youths so that change could occur in the school environment to support what the group was attempting to accomplish.

These youths need to see what they are doing and to gain some satisfaction from group activities. In structuring group activities which would enhance self-concepts, it was decided with the members' permission to organize the group as a club with officers, dues, weekly meetings, activities, and discussion of problems. For many of these youths, even assuming the role of an officer in a club was a new experience, one they faced with trepidations and anxieties. Some members laughed at early efforts—"jived* around a great deal"—but in time, this behavior decreased as group members provided support to the officers and gave recognition to other group members who attempted to involve themselves in group activities. The "jockeying"** for positions of power and influence initially was problematic but eventually greater cooperation presented itself as members gained security and could call each other on unproductive behavior.

The tuning-in phase was directed at securing information on how the members viewed the school, what they felt were problem areas, and what they wanted from the group. In the early phases of group development, members encountered difficulties in identifying and discussing their academic and behavioral problems and focused more on how the teachers were giving them problems. Discussions of how the situation might improve led to a recognition of academic problems, fears of being transferred to a special school, and some questioning of their abilities to do better. This knowledge led to the identification of a common ground and an identification of what the school and the group members could do to improve the situation. The school was willing to provide tutoring services and the students could admit that they could use some help in improving their school work. The group members agreed (contract establishment) that they would attempt to improve academically and behaviorally. The work phase was characterized by members' offering assistance to each other, planning of group activities, reading minutes, giving reports, discussion of areas of concern, and planning for the "bash" at termination.

At the termination stage, the group membership was approximately 15; some members dropped out, but returned on occasions; a couple were transferred to a special school. During the existence of the group, some members were expelled and some continued to be sent to the principal's office. However, the group was definitely a

---

*Jiving is a form of communication which basically lacks substance; it is flattering in nature and is directed at influencing the image of group members or manipulating the worker. It is cunning in nature.

**Jockeying is a form of promoting alliances, establishing cliques, gaining power, and recognition through establishing roles within the group. It is basically a process of establishing positions within the group and is similar to the power and control stage of Garland and Kolodny (1981).

progressive force. The school was satisfied with the group and what it was accomplishing, and along with the members, expressed the wish that the group would resume in the fall. For the members, the group met a kind of social hunger in which they gained acceptance and validation as individuals of worth. Brief highlights of two group sessions will reveal group interactions and how these interactions provided a transforming experience for these youths.

Session #3

Frank, age 14, had been elected as the secretary. Initially, he rejected this office but decided to accept it following much support from the group. At this meeting Frank was asked to read the minutes of the previous meeting. (At session #2, Frank stated he did not know how to take minutes, but valiantly made an attempt.) It was obvious Frank was extremely nervous, could not make out some words, and hesitated in his reading. The anxiety was added to by group members' "signifying." (This is a form of teasing which ends in the object of the "signifying" becoming angry.) Frank became angry, threw the minutes on the floor, and a confrontation appeared imminent. I expressed the opinion that I knew Frank could do it, that it wasn't too cool to laugh at people who were trying. I asked if anyone could do better. The members were silent, and I stated, "See Frank, no one can do better. Why don't you try it again?" With support Frank picked up the minutes and began to read again. This time there was silence and no horsing around. When Frank finished, I clapped and soon other members joined in. "See Frank," I said, "I knew you could do it."

Session #12

I asked where Frank was, as he had missed several meetings. John (in his usual role of spokesman) stated Frank was expelled. He got into trouble with Mr. Smith (a teacher). John stated Mr. Smith was a bad dude and this refrain was picked up by several group members. (The term "bad dude" can have negative or positive connotations.) Mr. Smith shoved Frank following an argument as he was taking him to the principal's office. Frank was sent home. Several members felt this was it for Frank, and that even though he was trying it didn't pay off and he would be sent to a special school.

I showed my anger that this would happen and I was not informed. I stated I would look into this and report back to the group next week. Then I asked questions about this "bad dude, Mr. Smith." John stated he didn't like Blacks, was always hassling them and no one liked him. I suggested maybe Mr. Smith should be invited to our next meeting to let him know their feelings. Silence pervaded the session. I asked, "Who wanted to invite him?" No one volunteered. As a measure of support, I stated I would be at the meeting. I looked at Robert, smiled slightly. Robert got the message and stated with an air of toughness that he would do it.

INSIGHTS GAINED FROM THE GROUP/GENERAL APPLICABILITY TO GROUP WORK WITH BLACKS

The group experience with low-income Black youths demonstrated that Blacks can benefit from group experiences and that self-concepts, social competencies, and psychosocial-educational skills can be enhanced for this population through the use of the small group. This group experience provided some practice-wisdom and insights which the author thinks has applicability for group work with Blacks in general.

1. The focus of group work with Blacks must be directed at the enhancement of self-concepts, improving coping skills, and the gaining of a sense of empowerment. Attention must be placed on the transactions which occur between Blacks and social systems. The group should not be viewed as a psychotherapeutic one in which objectives are to rehabilitate Blacks to conform to dehumanizing social systems. The dual focus (individual and society) is imperative.
2. The group worker must view and evaluate members' behavior in light of their experiences in American society. Low-income Black youths will present behavior which fluctuates between maturity, immaturity, and pseudomaturity.
3. Action-oriented techniques are more suited to the needs of Blacks rather than intellectual discussions or insight-oriented

processes. Group members must be able to see what they are doing (activities) as well as the benefits/outcomes which result from these activities.

4. The group leader will need to be able to accept anger and to use humor in diffusing some heavy situations, particularly those in which a member may present almost uncontrollable anger. (Blacks have often used humor as a survival technique.)

5. The group worker must be comfortable in self-disclosures and must be able to enter into the world of Blacks.

6. The group worker will serve as a model and will assume an active role in providing guidance and direction. Thus, the group will inevitably contain an educational component.

7. Race is a variable which presents itself in a covert or overt manner and must be addressed. Racism permeates all areas of Blacks' interactions with social systems, consciously or unconsciously. Racism has negatively affected Blacks' self-concepts, influenced their attitudes and behavior, and has contributed to a sense of powerlessness. In this sense, it is more appropriate to have a Black to serve as the group worker since he/she has a more accurate understanding of what these youths have experienced and the odds which they must overcome. A white group worker lacking this knowledge may focus more on the need for modification of behavior for assimilative purposes instead of racial validation and the development of social competencies which will enhance self-concepts.

8. The group worker on occasions must be confrontative. The confrontation is always posed as a challenge, never in a put-down or punitive manner: "I don't know if you can do better. You keep talking but nothing happens."

9. Physical contacts with group members should be carefully evaluated, particularly with low-income Black youths. Physical contacts may contain "sexual connotations," such as the person being "funny." If abrupt, they may remind these youths of past experiences with adults in which authority was implemented in a negative manner.

10. The group worker must be wary of providing direct advice. Low-income Black youths are always being advised or admonished about something and have built up much resistance toward advice which is transferred onto all adult figures.

11. Low-income Black youths do not always engage in direct eye contact and can reveal considerable feelings through their eyes. As a matter of fact, they frequently communicate through their eyes as verbal communication is sometimes uncomfortable to them and frequently may lead them into difficulties.
12. The group worker must be prepared for a prolonged period of challenging and testing before a relationship is established and even then the relationship will have a fragile quality and must constantly be reinforced.

CONCLUSIONS

Group work with low-income Black youths in the public school can be an effective form of intervention by which large numbers of low-income Black youths can be reached and helped to address the conditions which are negatively impacting on their education. These youths stand in need of positive psychosocial-educational experiences in which their self-concepts can be strengthened and their racial identities validated. The small group can accomplish this purpose. We think that Schwartz's reciprocal model and its theoretical underpinnings from systems theory and social psychology provides the group work model which is most applicable to group work with Blacks.

REFERENCES

Bank, J. A., and Grambs, J.D. (Eds.). *Black self-concept*, New York: McGraw-Hill, 1972.
Blumer, H. *Symbolic interactionism: Perspective and method*. Englewood Cliffs, NJ: Prentice-Hall, 1969.
Brayboy, T. The black patient in group therapy. *International Journal of Group Psychotherapy*, July, 1971, 288-293.
Bromley, D., and Longino, C. *White racism and black Americans*. Cambridge, MA: Schenkman Publishing Co., 1972.
Brown, J., and Arevalo, R. Group work with Chicano youths: The multi-model perspective. Paper presented at Second Annual Symposium Social Work with Groups, Arlington, University of Texas, 1980.
Challenging the Myths: The Schools, the Blacks and the Poor. Harvard Educational Review, Reprint Series #5, Second Printing, 1973.
Fisher, C. *Minorities, civil rights and protest*. Belmont, CA: Dickinson Publishing Co., 1970.
Garland, J., and Kolodny, R. *The treatment of children through social group work: A developmental approach*. Boston: Charles River Books, 1981.

Glasser, P., Sarri, R., and Vinter, R. (Eds.). *Individual change through small groups.* New York: Free Press, 1974.
Hartford, M. *Groups in social work.* New York: Columbia University Press, 1971.
Helping people in groups. Washington, D.C.: U.S. Dept. of Health, Education and Welfare, 1965.
Katz, I. Academic motivation and equal educational opportunity. *Harvard Educational Review*, Winter, 1960, p. 56-65.
Klein, A. *Effective group work.* New York: Association Press, 1972.
Logan, S.L. Race, identity and black children: A developmental perspective. *Social Casework*, January, 1981, p. 47-56.
Long, J. T., *Why we feel and behave as we do: A minority perspective.* West Covina, CA: John T. Long Publishing Co., 1975.
Papell, C., and Rothman, B. Social group work models: Possession and heritage. *Journal of Education for Social Work*, Fall, 1966, p. 66-77.
Pearson, R. Working with the disadvantaged through groups. *Counseling the Disadvantaged Youth*, William Amos and Jean Dresden Grambs. Englewood Cliffs, NJ: Prentice-Hall, 1968.
Potentials for service through groups in public welfare. Chicago, American Public Welfare Association, 1962.
Poussaint, A., and Atkinson, C. Black youth and motivation. *Race Relations: Current Perspectives*, Edgar E. Eps, (Ed.). Cambridge, MA: Winthrop Publishers, Inc., 1973.
Rist, R.C. Student social class and teacher expectation: The self-fulfilling prophecy in ghetto education. *Challenging the Myths: The Schools, the Blacks and the Poor*, Cambridge, MA: *Harvard Educational Review*, Reprint Series #5, Second Printing, 1973.
Schwartz, W. Social group work: The interactionist approach. *Encyclopedia of Social Work*, ed., John B. Turner, Vol. 2, New York, National Association of Social Workers, 1977, pp. 1328-1338.
Shulman, L. *The Skills of Helping: Individuals and Groups.* Itasca, IL: Peacock Publishers, 1979.
Strauss, A. *Mirrors and masks: The search for identity.* Glencoe, IL: Free Press, 1959; Reprinted Sociology Press, USA, 1969.
Roberts, R., and Northen, H. *Theories of social work with groups.* New York: Columbia University Press, 1976.
Whittaker, J. Models of group development: Implications for social group work practice. *The Practice of Social Work*, eds., Robert Klenk and Robert M. Ryan, Second Edition, Belmont, CA: Wadsworth Publishing Co., 1974.
Yinger, J.M. *A minority group in American society.* New York: Random House, 1964.

Group Work with Black Adoptive Applicants

Ruth G. McRoy
Zena Oglesby

ABSTRACT. The variety of uses of groups in the field of adoptions is traced historically and the group process is presented as an effective approach to studying prospective adoptive families. A case study of a culturally specific group of prospective black adoptive applicants is described and analyzed. Special emphasis is placed on the unique skills and knowledge needed by adoption workers in establishing trust and relationships with groups of black families who are interested in adopting.

USE OF GROUPS IN ADOPTION

Group methods have been employed during all phases of the adoption process from intake to post adoption follow-up services. Initially, groups were designed to offer an effective and efficient means of introducing prospective parents to the procedures, policies, eligibility criteria, etc. of adoption agencies (Wiehe, 1972). Such orientation groups were often used to weed out those prospective applicants who were not eligible to adopt, according to specified agency guidelines. Generally these agencies were primarily concerned with placing the "ideal adoptable child" the white healthy infant, for whom the demand was great, but the supply limited. The actual screening process of prospective families was accomplished through individual interviews with parents.

Post-placement adoptive parent discussion groups were introduced in many adoption agencies during the '50s in order to (1) pro-

---

Ruth G. McRoy, PhD, is Assistant Professor, School of Social Work, University of Texas at Austin, Austin, TX. Zena Oglesby, MSW, is Assistant Instructor, School of Social Work, University of Texas at Austin, Austin, TX.

mote discussion and mutual support among families who had finalized the adoption and (2) provide an effective means to supplement the worker's post placement supervisory visits to the family prior to finalization. For example, between 1955 and 1966, Louise Wise Services in New York City, held about 50 such groups representing some 500 couples. Their experiences revealed that many families, even years after the finalization of the adoption, continued to need an opportunity to share their joys as well as frustrations about adoptive parenthood. This represented a shift from the earlier position of adoption experts that agency communication with adoptive parents after the adoption is finalized tends to promote dependency on the agency (Biskind, 1966, p. 562). Group experiences have been found to be very appropriate means of bolstering parental security through discussions on infertility and on suggested approaches for informing the child of the circumstances which led to his or her adoption (p. 564).

By the 1960s a few adoption agencies had begun considering the use of groups not only at intake or during post placement, but as an integral part of the adoption process. The group approach represented a radical departure from the traditional casework adoption evaluation called the "adoption home study." This often consists of an intake interview, a series of three to six joint and individual sessions, a home evaluation, and final interview. If there are children or other family members residing in the home, they too are generally interviewed. Questions which focus on the couple's motivation for adoption, feelings about infertility (if appropriate), or financial status may be addressed. Any educative or anxiety reduction activities are primarily dependent upon the skill and inclination of the individual social worker. At the culmination of the study, a fairly lengthy evaluative report of the home study is prepared, and applicants are notified of their acceptance or rejection.

In the mid-1960s a Lutheran agency in Washington, D.C., decided to experiment with group adoptive home studies. A caseworker (observer) and group worker conducted four weekly group meetings for prospective parents. Interviews with references were held and the caseworker made an individual home visit. Each couple was asked to write an autobiography and complete a medical history and application form (Dillow, 1968, p. 151).

As the group discussions covered the same topics as in any home study (feelings about fertility, competition with biological parents, expectations of the child, etc.), the group worker and caseworker found that the group process provided an effective means to lessen anxiety and facilitate mutual sharing about their questions related to becoming adoptive parents.

By the late 1960s and early 1970s, many adoption agencies were expanding their services to recruit families for school age, minority, and physically or emotionally handicapped children. Cognizant that families for such children needed special preparation, many agencies found the group process to be particularly effective in working with prospective applicants. In 1967, Middlestadt et al. reported that Lutheran Social Services in Wichita, Kansas, had begun using group orientations as a beginning step in preparing applicants for parenthood (p. 365). Operating under the assumption that the agency expected to be able to place a child with all who applied, Lutheran Social Services used the introductory group interview with four to eight couples as the first stage in the adoption preparation process. Couples were informed about the adoption process, given application forms, and encouarged to share their common concerns about becoming adoptive parents. The subsequent sessions with applicants also were designed to prepare them for receiving a child and becoming a family (p. 377).

Similarly, the Maine Children's Home for Little Wanderers set up group sessions which included a series of films, lectures, homework assignments, and discussions about the children available for adoption. The group atmosphere provided a combination of an educative and screening function for applicants (Goodridge, 1975, p. 35-39).

Other agencies have utilized both extended group studies as well as marathon studies for prospective adoptive parents. For example, Lutheran Family and Children's Services in St. Louis offered families a choice between an intensive group experience lasting from nine to 20 hours over a specified block of time or an extended group lasting for five consecutive weeks or alternate weeks. Both groups were designed to prepare applicants for parenthood and were used in conjunction with at least one individual interview which focused on the couples' specific request for a child and other unresolved issues or concerns noted during the group process (Wiehe, 1972, p. 646).

Overall, most adoption agencies have found that group approaches tend to facilitate both the goals of preparation for adoptive parenthood and evaluation of prospective adoptive parents. The group experience has been found to be cost-effective, tends to improve worker-client communication during and following placement, and educates adoptive applicants about the needs of "hard to place children" (Wiehe, 1972; Anderson and Kaufman, 1973, p. 51).

THE TREMETIERE MODEL

In 1972 Tressler-Lutheran Service Associates in York, Pennsylvania, designed a "client-centered" group approach for evaluating prospective adoptive couples. According to this model, groups of five to seven couples or single applicants meet together for approximately nine sessions. Through the process, adoption exchange books are available to enable families to become cognizant of the kinds of children available. A panel of adoptive parents are brought in for two group sessions and are asked to talk about their experiences with adoption. Also, prospective adoptive families visit the homes of families who have already adopted the type of child the applicants wish to adopt.

The group members participate in value clarification exercises and discuss the use of Transactional Analysis and Parent Effectiveness Training in enhancing interaction and communication skills with children. They complete "feeling autobiographies, health forms, and thought sheets" on each session. At the culmination, the agency staff check references, visit homes, and record their impressions. Thus, the family's life study is basically written by the parents for presentation to agencies (Tremetiere, 1979, p. 683).

Between 1972 and 1979, the Tressler-Lutheran Agency placed over 1000 children in adoptive homes and reported a 95 percent success rate (p. 683). Advocating this new group study method, Barbara Tremetiere, the agency's Adoption Program Director, toured the West Coast between 1978 and 1979. San Bernadino (California) County adoption workers were particularly intrigued by this new approach and quickly established several groups of white adoptive applicants.

FORMING A BLACK ADOPTIVE APPLICANTS GROUP

About two weeks after the first San Bernadino County adoptive study groups were underway, the agency received calls from five black families who expressed an interest in adopting. Two adoption workers decided to try using the Tremetiere approach with these families. Neither the black male worker nor the white female had any prior group experience with adoptive parents.

Due to the limited number of black adoptive applicants at the time, all five, regardless of background characteristics, were considered potential candidates for the group. Applicants were interviewed individually in their homes. The black worker conducted each of these sessions in order to facilitate the establishment of trust and to give support and encouragement to the applicants. This was considered critical in order to increase the likelihood that the applicants would complete the home study process.

To encourage each family to be open in expressing feelings of anxiety, apprehension, or distrust, the social worker conducted the interview without note taking or recording equipment. Each of the couples asked questions about the format for the group process and wanted clarification regarding the role the white social worker would play. All applicants seemed to initially fear that the white worker had the real decision-making power to approve their adoption application. They were reassured that both workers were equal in authority and that they were part of a team. The black worker insisted that he would be their advocate throughout the process. Although all the families were told that participation in the group was totally optional, none of the five families chose to withdraw or to participate in a traditional home study.

OVERVIEW OF THE GROUP PROCESS

Group Composition

The black adoptive parent's group consisted of five couples who ranged in age from middle twenties to late thirties. All had been married for at least five years, and both the husband and wife worked. The average family income ranged from $30,000 to $45,000. Among their diverse occupations were the following: laborer, beautician, teacher, social worker, and military. All but one had at least some college education and four applicants had college degrees. Three couples lived in urban areas and two in rural areas. All of the applicants were requesting children less than 8 years of age and were willing to accept mild handicaps.

Group meetings were scheduled for two and one half hours on

Wednesday evenings for a period of eight weeks. Several couples drove as much as three hours from the upper-California desert to attend the meetings. The San Bernadino County Credit Union was selected as the meeting site because it was considered a neutral location, easily accessible, and having adequate parking.

Group Process

This group adhered to the format and content employed in Tremetiere groups. During two of the group sessions several single and married adoptive parents visited the group to share their experiences with adoption.

Group members had to complete written homework which included self-analysis assignments and a comprehensive autobiography. As several of the group members had difficulty in expressing themselves in writing, a policy was instituted which allowed anyone to record his or her autobiography on cassette tape and later have it transcribed by the agency clerical staff. This action served to assure group members that the agency was flexible and sincerely interested in assisting them in their efforts to become adoptive parents rather than creating barriers.

Participants displayed some resistance in utilizing the Parent Effectiveness Training as they disagreed with the emphasis on extensive parent/child negotiation and the prohibition against corporal punishment. As all but two of these prospective adoptive couples were already raising children, they felt that they had already developed effective discipline techniques and felt that the PET principles were not needed. Furthermore, some participants felt that PET did not reflect "black values in child rearing." This concern was resolved by spending one session discussing and evaluating disciplinary approaches currently in use by participants and when appropriate, suggesting alternatives.

Similarly, the role play component of the Termetiere approach, was not well received either. Group members seemed very uncomfortable with this activity and verbalized a feeling that this was "childish." However, rather than abandoning the entire program, workers altered the approach. For example, the active listening concept was removed from the role play situation. Instead the black worker gave examples of active listening from his own experiences with his wife and encouraged feedback and experience sharing from the participants. Prospective adoptive parents were asked to practice active listening at home with their mates and, in later sessions, the worker explained the significance of this exercise to problems encountered in communicating with children. The approach seemed to be useful as a means for teaching parenting techniques for raising adopted school age children.

Social Worker Roles

Both social workers found that they had to assume the role of group members first and group facilitators second. Many participants were distrustful of the agency and the adoption process. Most were aware of other black families who had applied to adopt through adoption agencies but for some reason had never received a child. Consequently, these prospective black adoptive couples seemed to place a great deal of emphasis on trust and cohesiveness within the group. Group members felt that the loyalty of the workers was exemplified by their willingness to share their own feelings and personal experiences within the group and serving as advocates on behalf of each member's interest in adopting a child.

Distrust of the ''welfare department'' was verbalized openly and often and the worker's response was used as a barometer of how much he or she could be trusted. Throughout the group experience the social workers found that they had to convince the participants that they would intercede for the prospective parents, if they were not treated fairly by the agency. However, the workers repeatedly informed the group that their overriding allegiance and concern focused on the best interests of the black children for whom homes were being sought.

At the onset of the group, little interaction took place between the white worker and the group. The members perceived the white worker to be their evaluator and the black worker as their advocate. However, well into the second group meeting, each member was asked to tell something that was unique about himself or herself. When the white worker described in a very comical manner her escapades as a bird watcher, the entire group laughed hysterically. Almost instantaneously, this self-disclosure of a very humorous experience seemed to release the tensions and anxieties within the group toward the one non-black participant. In each succeeding session the white worker began to feel accepted as a full-fledged member of the group and the entire group seemed to coalesce.

Group Culture

These upwardly mobile black group members were similar in a variety of ways. All had experienced some degree of racism, had family ties in the south, strong education, and achievement orientation for themselves and their children. All but one couple had an extended family support system and some form of parenting experience. Three of the ten participants had attended the same school system in Louisiana and shared the experiences of being born and reared in the same southern state.

The workers emphasized that this group represented the agency's first attempt at a group home study for black adoptive families. As a result the group developed a very strong sense of pride and group identity characteristic of "first cohorts." For example, phone numbers and addresses were exchanged at the first group meeting. This group cohesion remained intact long after each couple had received a child. Only one of the ten participants ever missed a session and this particular member had her husband tape the group session for her. Moreover, several years later the group formed the nucleus of a black adoptive parent advocacy group.

At the culmination of the group sessions, one couple withdrew their application to adopt after admitting to the worker that the husband was an alcoholic. They acknowledged that the group experience forced them to recognize that they needed professional help before they could consider adopting a child. Explaining that they had felt a true sense of belonging in the group, the couple hesitated, however, to withdraw their adoption application until the group sessions were over.

Termination

The group chose to have a family barbeque at a member's home during the last group meeting. This session was used by the participants to officially declare the workers as friends and to cement contacts between group members. Many expressed a great deal of separation anxiety as they knew that they were about to lose contact with persons who had become personal friends. This feeling was particularly intense among the couples who lived in the California desert and resided about three-hours driving distance from the other families. Another factor which tended to exaggerate group members concerns about separation was that they each had to individually complete the adoption process and await a child. To make this experience less stressful, the families agreed to remain in regular telephone contact with one another. At this final meeting, the group reflected on their experiences over the past eight weeks and agreed that they probably would never have completed the adoption process had they not had the group's support. They predicted that, without the group sessions, the individual home study would probably have been disastrous for them as it had been for many of their acquaintances. One of the five husbands in this group stated: "I would not have been as open about my feelings and ideas in an individual interview, especially had it taken place in the agency's office. It would have felt like I was sitting in a police station." Finally, it was suggested that the number of group study sessions be expanded.

DISCUSSION

Cultural differences must be taken into consideration in conducting studies of prospective black adoptive families. Adoptive applicants generally feel extremely vulnerable knowing they are to be judged on their potential parenting capabilities (Herzog, p. 16). Many black families fail to even initiate or complete the adoption process as they tend to fear such a judgmental process (Day, p. 68).

The experience in this group and subsequent groups provided evidence that the race and attitude of the social worker were important variables in determining group cohesion and establishing a trusting relationship with group leaders. Having a black male worker serve as a role model and group facilitator was a critical element in this group process. Moreover, the worker's willingness to share his own experiences with the group promoted trust.

The participants in this group felt that they could relate easily to a black worker because "he has been there and understands." From the experiences of this group, the ideal group co-leaders would be a black male and female. If this is not possible due to the limited number of black social workers in the adoption field, having one black and one white as co-leaders (preferably male and female) would be a viable option.

CONCLUSION

Within two years of the completion of this first black adoptive parent group home study, all four couples who completed the process received children. They have become adoption advocates and maintain close relationships with each other.

Since mid-1979, nine all-black group home studies have been conducted in San Bernadino county. These groups comprised approximately 90 participants (couples and singles). Of this total, ten individuals have dropped out of the process (four couples and two singles) resulting in an 89 percent retention rate. Of those black families approved for adoption, only one has opted to adopt outside the county system (private agency) and all other have now received children.

From the foregoing statistics of completed group adoptive home studies of black families, it is obvious that this approach is very effective. Among the advantages of this approach are the following:

(1) The group home study gives applicants an opportunity to interact with others like themselves, who have expressed an interest in adopting a black child. Applicants can share their concerns and anxieties and achieve identification with others in an atmosphere of mutual support.

(2) The group interaction serves to reduce isolation and fosters the development of support systems external to the adoption agency. Such networks may lead to formalized adoption advocacy and support groups, such as those formed in California.

(3) Interest in adoptive parenting is increased through the group process by educating and shattering myths about adoption. Consequently, many of the participants were willing not only to adopt themselves, but be active in recruiting other black families to adopt through the agency.

(4) Through the group experience, agencies can prepare prospective adoptive parents for the realities of raising children from often difficult and diverse background experiences.

(5) The self-esteem of applicants may be raised as a by-product of the group experience. Prospective adoptive families not only learn about the intricacies of raising school age children, but have an opportunity to learn about themselves, to realistically examine their own lives, and acknowledge their strengths and limitations. The natural support from group members along with the support of the worker tends to be ego-nourishing and serves to improve self-images of the applicants.

(6) Through group home studies, more applicants can be studied in a shorter period of time and thus increase the number of approved black families available for the thousands of black children needing adoptive homes.